"Excuse Me, Doctor! I've Got What?"

"Excuse Me, Doctor! I've Got What?"

*Taking Ownership of Your Health and
Making Healthcare Reform Work for You*

Melissa E. Clarke, MD

The information in this book does not replace the advice of a medical professional. It is not the intent of the author to diagnose or prescribe through this book. The intent is only to offer information to help you work with your doctor in your mutual quest for desirable health. Any application of the recommendations set forth in the following pages is at the reader's discretion. The reader should consult with his or her own physician concerning the recommendations in this book. In addition, medical knowledge is constantly changing as new information becomes available. The author has, as far as it is possible, taken care to ensure that the information given in this text is accurate and up-to-date. However, readers are strongly advised to consult with their healthcare professional to confirm that the information complies with latest legislation and standards of practice.

This book was printed in the United States of America.

Rev. date: 01/08/2014

To order additional copies of this book, contact:
Xlibris LLC
1-888-795-4274
www.Xlibris.com
Orders@Xlibris.com
128738

THIS BOOK IS dedicated to my mentors and the multitude of patients who have given me the opportunity to practice the healing arts as well as earn their trust. In addition, my eternal gratitude goes to all who contributed to this book - Celeste Garcia, Phyllis Perry, and Eraka Rouzorondu for your review, words of wisdom and invaluable input; to Beryl Anderson West, Max Anderson, Marv West, Aungelique Proctor Anderson, Victor Freeman, and Stephanie Morton for your practical advice; and to the Brandonista, Tynisha Brooks, for her creative cover genius. I especially thank my mother Dr. Catherine Clarke and father Rupert Clarke, whose boundless love is my foundation. And to my wonderful husband, Wayne Bruce, the soul of understanding and love, thank you for supporting me in all I do.

CONTENTS

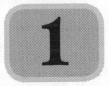

Introduction – Don't Be Blindsided

"**R**OOM 1'S GLUCOSE is off the charts! It wasn't responding to IV fluids alone, but it came down nicely with IV insulin. He'll need to come in – floor or ICU depending on his lab work."

"Room 2 – unbelievable, but part of her left breast is eroded from cancer, and it is now infected. She is a recent immigrant from Kenya, and she didn't go to the doctor because she had no way to afford it. It may be too late if the cancer has spread, but she'll definitely need to be admitted for antibiotics, surgical resection, and an oncology consult . . ."

"Room 3 – teenager admitted for asthma exacerbation, just waiting for a bed upstairs. He was playing ball and didn't want to stop until he was just about not breathing. We almost had to intubate him on arrival, but he has cleared up significantly after Epi, Solumedrol, and continuous nebulizers. He is still going to pediatric ICU, though . . ."

These were just three of the many patients I discussed with the doctor relieving me after a typical night in an urban emergency department in the heart of Washington DC. As the admitting emergency physician, I often wondered how these individuals would do once they got their immediate crisis resolved. Leaving the hospital was just the beginning of their journey. Living successfully day to day with the challenge of their illness, and getting good quality care was really what they had to master . . .

Why This Book?

"Excuse me, Doctor! I've got *what?*"

When the shock wears off, when the reality settles in, when someone is diagnosed with a chronic illness, what do they do about it?

Navigating today's medical care is like being put in the middle of a forest with no compass and having to find your way through it. The potential twists, turns, and dead ends are numerous. And the stakes are high because we are dealing with our own health, our most precious resource.

As a doctor working in a large inner-city emergency department, I often saw the consequences of people trying to navigate blindly on their own. People ended up in the ER for multiple reasons that could have been avoided if they were adequately equipped or even had a guide to help them through. Reasons ranged from having no primary doctor to lacking health insurance to having no knowledge about caring for their condition . . . and the list goes on and on. There are hundreds of cracks in our health system, and it is incredibly easy for anyone using it to fall into one of them. Adding to the confusion are the changes now occurring because of health-care reform. They are all well intentioned and will ultimately improve the quality of health care provided. However, in the interim, regular people feel confused and uncertain about how health-care reform will affect their daily experience with their health-care provider, their ability to access care when they need it, and their pocketbook.

I wrote this book to serve as a guide for any patient who has used our health-care system and felt lost, vulnerable, and frustrated. Even I, as a doctor, have had these feelings as I have witnessed firsthand how frustrating it can be to get high-quality care for myself and my loved ones. I have learned, though, that it does not have to be this way. I came to that conclusion through years of working in multiple areas of health care, and personal experience as a patient and caregiver. In addition, I have seen how the changes brought about by health-care reform will affect you and how you can best prepare for it and make it work to your advantage. My goal is to share these strategies so you can actually be empowered when it comes to your health-care experience. This book is a comprehensive resource for patient empowerment that gives practical, in-depth, holistic information that prepares any reader to navigate the American health-care system *and* manage the emotional and physical experiences of having a chronic health condition. It is intended to set you up to take charge of your health and be the best advocate for yourself and your loved ones.

Our Changing Health-Care System

Are you ready for the changes being brought about by health-care reform? Do many readers even know what they are and how they will affect you? Here is the scoop in a nutshell.

Health care touches the lives of nearly everyone in the United States – from being born in a hospital, to living as a senior in an assisted living facility, and everything in between. Whether you obtain medical insurance through your employer, seek consultation with a doctor about an illness, fill a prescription at the pharmacy, try a chiropractor for back pain – almost everyone rubs elbows with the U.S. health-care system.

But this health-care system is changing rapidly. Here is why change is happening. We as Americans have been using the health-care system more than ever before. The reasons are multiple and include increasing exposure to environmental chemicals, an aging population, couch-potato/desk-potato lifestyles, and less nutrient-rich diets. The overall result is that the number of people needing ongoing treatment for what we call chronic disease – like diabetes, heart failure, multiple sclerosis, dementia, and strokes – is growing dramatically. As the number of people needing health care has increased, so have health-care costs. These costs are growing so rapidly that in a few years, we, individually and as a country, will not be able to afford them. And even though we pay more now than ever before to get care, we still do not know if each time we go to the doctor or hospital, we are getting the best, or even good, quality care.

These forces led to health-care reform and the Affordable Care Act (ACA), also called Obamacare. The ACA has several components to address many of our system's cracks. The first is through reforms that improve access to insurance – young adults being on their parents' medical policy until age twenty-six, preventing insurance companies from denying coverage for those with preexisting conditions, and setting up insurance exchanges so individuals can get low-cost health insurance. A second component is improving access to medical care through provisions like funding community health centers, where people can get low-cost care, and helping seniors with the cost of medicines. Very importantly, the ACA also addresses the quality of medical care doctors and hospitals are providing. The quality of care changes are designed to reward health-care providers when they focus efforts on keeping patients well and out of the hospital instead of getting paid mostly when people are sick and in the hospital. Under health-care reform, doctors get rewarded for the quality of the care they give and how well their patients are doing, not just the number of procedures and office visits they perform. There are also parts of the ACA that pay for research to help doctors know which treatments have the best and safest results.

But this is the kicker – a huge portion of containing costs in health care will be put squarely on the shoulders of health consumers themselves. This may come as a surprise to many and blindside others. Each of us will be expected to assume a greater role in our own health care. The new buzz word is "promoting self-care," which essentially means that each person will be expected to get health insurance, know all about their own health and health conditions, take their medicines, go regularly to the doctor (since the issue of getting health insurance and affording care will be out of the way), choose cost-effective treatments and providers, and successfully navigate the system. In some instances, those who do not adopt this perspective will likely have some financial penalty to face or miss out on some financial reward. Essentially, you will be expected to be the owner of your health-care experience.

This book is a manual to guide you through all the changes that are expected of you. It provides the tools to assist you in getting the best care for yourself and your loved ones in these rapidly changing times. Taking ownership of your health-care experience requires several steps. We will cover each of them in depth in the chapters to come.

How to Use This Book

Think of this book as a manual to equip you to take ownership of your health-care experience. Every chapter has practical information you can apply to affect your health-care experience. The end of each chapter contains "Takeaway Checklists," which summarize the information presented in an easily accessible format. Starting in chapter 2, we address the huge shift that is taking place in how we think about our own roles and the role of our doctor. Our personal doctor has traditionally been the one to have all the say in our care, a kind of one-way relationship in which we passively received care. But that model has changed, and now a new model exists where we are actually the central player – the quarterback, if you will – in our health-care decisions. In this new scenario, we will review what tools and strategies you have at your disposal for your new role as the central player on your health-care team. In chapters 3 and 4, we discuss the steps in taking control of what you can influence yourself. We will review actions you can take to understand and promote your own health, no matter what your health condition is. We will then cover all the steps involved in getting high-quality, affordable care that is right for you and your family. This first involves choosing your health-care team – understanding who all the various players are (chapter 5) – and then how to pick the right ones and form effective working relationships with them (chapters 6 and 7). You will then know how to choose and effectively work with a health professional partner, whether it be a conventional doctor or alternative practitioner, the various healing techniques used, and which have proven effective for what ailments. Should you need a hospitalization, in chapter 8, we understand strategies on how to maximize the benefit of that stay and how to successfully transition out of the hospital back to home or wherever you will next receive care. Chapter 9 discusses how to decide if a clinical trial is right for you. And finally, in chapter 10, we discuss how to afford it all – how to find the financial and social resources to manage the costs of health care, whether it is alternative or conventional.

This book contains important general knowledge for everyone to have as they interact with the health-care system. However, just like any other manual, it is good to know what areas to refer to for which specific problems. Let us look at several different scenarios where you may be managing specific issues and want immediate answers from a specific section of this book.

- Newly interested in how to stay well and get a good professional partner in health to help you do so (general health maintenance) – chapters 3, 4, and 5 explain how we get sick, strategies to stay well, and how to choose the right health-care partners.
- Recently diagnosed with an illness – the majority of this book is intended just for you. With it, you can start to chart your course for your health-care journey fully prepared and

ready. Chapter 2 provides the tools for you to be emotionally ready for the journey. Chapters 3 through 6 explain how we get sick, strategies to stay well, and choosing health-care partners to help you do so. Chapter 9 helps you with the decision-making about being in a research trial for your condition. Chapter 10 helps with strategies to deal with the financial side of dealing with illness.

- Already diagnosed with a chronic illness but looking for new strategies to manage it and improve your health – you may already have chosen your doctor or have a great insurance plan, but you want to address a specific issue. You can choose from the exact chapters that address your need. Of particular interest may be when to get a second opinion (in chapter 7), considering a clinical trial (chapter 9), or how to get the most from your health insurance company (chapter 10).

- About to be hospitalized and need to know what to expect and how to best manage it – chapter 8 reviews all the strategies on making the most of your hospital stay and being prepared for successfully transitioning back home or to a rehabilitation facility.

Altogether, this how-to manual transforms you into a savvy consumer who can benefit from the wide array of options available for your care. You will not only gain information about how to better care for yourself and choose the right practitioner – conventional or alternative – but also gain an understanding of how our health-care system works. You will know effective ways to manage your relationship with your doctor, insurance company, and hospital. I wish you success in your journey toward better health care and, most importantly, better health.

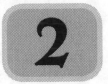

So You Are a Patient Now

If a person is treated like a patient,
they are apt to act like one.

– Frances Farmer

Paul was a gentleman I treated in the emergency room. The first time I saw him, it was for passing out and severe weakness. He turned out to have a super high blood sugar of over 900 – normal is between 60 and 100. This was the first time he heard the diagnosis of type 2 diabetes. He was admitted to the hospital for a few days, but I saw him right back again in the ER about three months later because of similar symptoms. Although his blood sugar was not as high as before, he was still pretty ill, and I asked him what was going on. He said he didn't understand why he had been feeling sick again because he had been taking his diabetes pills. The more I talked to him, though, the more it was clear he had no clue about his disease. He did not know what was required of him to be healthier, and he had never attended a diabetes education class. We set him up with an appointment for one before he went home from the ER. About a month later, I saw him in the hall after one of his visits with the certified diabetes nurse educator. "You know what, Doc?" he said. "I never knew what was going on with me. I thought that going to the doctor and taking my meds was enough to be OK. But Sheila, my diabetes nurse, showed me how I have been shooting myself in the foot and all the things I needed to do differently! Now I check my sugar four times a day, I watch what I eat, and I started walking a lot more! You know, now I feel so much better! I like you and all, but you don't ever have to worry about seeing me in the ER again!"

What Does Being a Patient Mean?

WHEN YOU ARE first diagnosed with an illness, you automatically become a patient. We rarely stop to think what does being a *patient* mean, and how does being a patient affect us moving forward and getting better.

The word *patient* originally meant "one who suffers." It comes from the related Latin and Greek words *patior* and *paskhein*, both meaning "suffering." Being ill can definitely feel like suffering. But at the same time, just the idea of the word "patient," one who suffers, puts us into a passive mind-set just like Paul had initially as a "diabetic patient." That passive patient mind-set can leave you feeling like you:

1. have no influence over what is happening to you – being told by your doctor, your nurse, or even your insurance company about your condition, your bills, and the medicines you have to take;
2. must be "patient" – waiting for the doctor, waiting for the X-ray result, waiting for the medicine to work – essentially waiting for help from the outside; and
3. must depend on a health-care provider of some sort to rescue you from what is happening.

This concept of patient mirrors exactly what the conventional doctor-patient relationship has been for a long time. Traditionally, from many doctors' standpoints, being a "good patient" means following exactly what the doctor says, preferably in an unquestioning manner. Our system is structured so that the power is put solely into the hands of the doctor to make it right. Often all decision making is blindly yielded to the doctor and the health-care system.

In some instances, this can work, and many people have been helped by this approach. However, there are many who have not been helped. This is why. First of all, being in the mind-set of "patient" may often mean not acknowledging your role in how you can affect your current health condition. There are very few chronic diseases for which there are external cures. The *chronic* in chronic disease means it does not go away or get cured because there is no medical treatment to make it go away. The most that medicine or surgery can do by itself in many instances is to keep you from dying from the illness or ending up in the hospital. It generally means that you can live with the disease but never get rid of it or, in the case of some cancers, always have the threat that it will return. Consumer trends reflect that people are starting to consider alternative healing systems since they are realizing that cures in conventional medicine do not exist for many conditions. However, it is important to realize that no magic bullet exists in any healing system. Even with alternative treatments like acupuncture or chiropractic, any improvements achieved will fade if you go back into the same patterns that gave rise to the problem in the first place. Changing those patterns to healthier ones is what can really affect the course of the disease and significantly improve your quality of life, just like Paul from the emergency room did with nutrition and exercise for diabetes. The take-home point is that having the best possible health requires a commitment to change and time to see the effect of those changes. Being in the mind-set of a traditional patient definitely does not prepare you to take this kind of approach to proactively manage your health.

The second reason that the word *patient* may not serve you well is that it may leave you more vulnerable to unintentional mistakes that can occur in the course of your care. Thousands of medical mistakes are made every year. Thousands more people die yearly as a result of these preventable medical errors than are killed in car crashes. Yet physicians and hospitals, until very recently, were largely unregulated. And conventional medicine is not the only place this happens. Punctured lungs can happen from acupuncture, spinal injuries from spinal manipulation, and fatal reactions can happen to herbal medicines – these occurrences are just less well documented. Even with the changes that health-care reform mandates to improve the quality of care, there is no guarantee that medical errors will be eliminated. Being a traditional patient who does not question your care or seek the safest and best possible treatments, raises the chances of being the recipient of poorer quality care and not getting the outcomes you want.

A Change in Perspective – Being an Empowered Health-Care Consumer

Own Your Health-Care Experience

Don't despair, though! I am not advocating trying to deal with health challenges solely on your own or that there is no use in getting medical care. Rather, the key is rather to adopt a different approach to your own health and change your perspective on how you go about getting health care. Rather than an entirely dependent relationship where we passively await help, we can instead adopt the mind-set of being a partner with our provider, where we take an active role in decisions that are being made. This automatically puts you as the patient into the front seat in being an active participant in your recovery. This is a huge change in perspective for many people, health-care users, and providers alike. This perspective is one that some health-care providers may not welcome (and those are the ones you should avoid). Being an active participant involves educating yourself about the condition you have, asking questions of your doctor, and advocating for yourself. Research shows that people with this approach, what I term an "empowered health-care consumer," get better results and are more satisfied with the care they get. These individuals are also less likely to report that they had an error with their medical care, medication, or lab tests. They actually have more positive views of the health system as a whole. Being empowered allows an individual to more easily make the changes necessary to shift out of the habits and choices that contributed to ill health in the first place. In addition, they can make better informed choices about the treatments they receive and how to live healthfully.

You Are Not Your Disease!

Another change in perspective involves not letting yourself be labeled as the disease that you currently have. It is common to hear providers and others refer to their patients as "the diabetic" or "the cancer patient." Some people even use this language to describe themselves – "I am an asthmatic" or "I am a diabetic." While you may currently have asthma or diabetes, it is a very subtle shift in attitude when you or someone else labels you as your disease. You start to define yourself and your identity as that disease. This thinking does not promote a shift to being well. Consider athletes training for an event. Athletes are taught to use visual imagery, a technique where they picture themselves successfully executing their plays or techniques. This mental imagery can take their game to the next level, thus giving them the mental edge to win. As an individual trying to deal with illness and trying to live "at the top of your game," you cannot gain a mental edge by thinking of yourself as "an asthmatic"; but you can picture yourself as someone with the tools and techniques to successfully manage and, in some cases, overcome the asthma condition that you have.

Get Educated

If you have gotten a new diagnosis, one of the most effective ways to become empowered is to educate yourself about your condition. The Internet has changed both the way individuals get medical information and, for many, the way they interact with doctors. A 2007 Pew Internet & American Life Project showed that people with disabilities and chronic conditions are more likely than others to look up health information. They then use that information and use that knowledge to ask their doctor questions or change the way they cope with a chronic condition. In the early days of the Internet, the American Medical Association actually asked that people not to go online for health information, both because there was little reliable information there at that time and because doctors were reluctant to give up their role as the primary source of health information. People started using the Internet and never looked back, though. Interestingly enough though, they are often hesitant to tell a doctor about what they find online because they do not want to be perceived as challenging their doctor.

Inaccurate information still abounds on the Internet. But an ever-growing number of people go there for health information and find great sources and resources to help them cope with, understand, and manage their condition. However, to be an informed, proactive health-care user, it is best for you or a loved one to seek out information and discuss this information with your health-care provider. Below are first some tips for finding accurate information.

How to Use the Internet to Self-Educate but Not Self-Diagnose

The Internet, while it has some great sources of health information, is not the best way to come up with a diagnosis. People who use the Internet to try to self-diagnose more often than not end up scaring themselves into thinking they have a life-threatening illness based on their symptoms. This is because they have no context for the information they read. There is even a term for it: *cyberchondria*, which is defined as "the excessive use of Internet health sites to fuel health anxiety" (really, it is a word!). I call it "medical student syndrome." My medical classmates and I, as well as medical students I have taught over the years, all thought that we had some life-threatening illness as we learned new diagnoses in medical school – thinking our sore throat was throat cancer or a tension headache was a brain hemorrhage. But after we gained experience and were able to put symptoms in context, that phase thankfully went away. The average lay person using the Internet for self-diagnosis is also likely to get alarmed and think that a symptom is indicative of a worst-case scenario. That is not to say true stories do not exist of individuals ending up having a diagnosis they found on the Internet. However, using the Internet in this way is often more anxiety provoking than accurate and productive.

Better uses of the Internet are to learn more about a health condition you already have or find resources to better cope with or treat your symptoms or condition. But first, you have to determine whether the website you are getting your information from is reliable. To that end, here are a few tips for Internet health investigating:

- **Who put up the site?** The responsible party behind the site can go a long way to helping you figure out if the information can be trusted. The "About Us" page tells you if the site is put up by a trusted information source such as a branch of the government (.gov), a university (.edu), or a nonprofit organization (.org). Examples of these would include the websites of the Mayo Clinic and the National Institutes of Health. While a business or commercial entity (.com) can provide reliable information, it is best to keep in mind that if there is a profit motive, claims may be embellished. It is always good to double-check information from these sources. Websites published by individuals may offer support and advice about coping with certain conditions and treatments. However, it's very important to double-check recommendations you see on a website published by an individual. Make sure they are references for the claims and discuss it with a health-care provider before trying it.

- **Is the information reviewed before it is posted?** Another quality check is to see if the site has an editorial board and if those members are experts in their field. There might be a section called "About Our Writers" or "About Our Authors." You can review this section to find out who has written the information and what their credentials are.

- **Where does the site get its information from?** Any website that provides health-related information should tell you the information's source. If it is not original to the person or organization that runs the website, the original source should be clearly stated. The original source should be one that provides unbiased information based on *research*. Also, for sites with advertisers, make sure that the source of health advice on the page is not the same as the advertisers. For example, if a page about treatment of headache recommends one therapy by name, see if you can tell if the company that makes the therapy is the one behind the page. If it is, you should consult other sources to see what they say about the same treatment.

- **Is the information outdated**? Medical knowledge is expanding rapidly. Just twenty years ago, the total body of medical knowledge took seven years to double; it now doubles in about seventy days. This rapid increase of knowledge makes it extremely important to know whether what you are reading is up to date. One way to do this is to check for a copyright line or date of last review, generally at the bottom of the page. Documents that propose to discuss the latest treatment or diagnosis of a condition should be reviewed at least yearly. However, a document on coping with the loss of a loved one does not need to be as current. In addition, explore the links on the site. Sites with a lot of broken links probably are not kept up to date.

- **Be suspicious of "miracle cures."** We have all seen the websites claiming quick, dramatic, or miraculous health results. One remedy will cure a variety of illnesses, or a breakthrough product or secret ingredient. They often use a sensational writing style and more than likely are not legitimate. The miracle cures are often not based on true scientific research. Instead, they rely on opinion in the form of testimonials from a few anonymous individuals, like "David from Tennessee." Look for legitimacy by checking for contact information on the people providing testimonials. Also, check more than one site to see if this is the only one making these claims.

- **Can the average person understand the content?** If the words and writing style on the site are deliberately obscure, scientific-sounding language, or jargon, beware. A health website for consumers should use simple language, not technical language.

- **Does the site tell you what they do with the information they collect?** Health information should always be confidential. If there is a registration form asking for personal information that could identify you, refer to the site's privacy policy. This link, "Privacy" or "Privacy Policy," should tell you if your information is really being protected or, if not, what the company is doing with it. For example, if the site says "We share information with companies that can provide you with useful products," then your information isn't private.

- **Consult with your health professional**. Last, but not least, if you are ever unsure about information you get from the Internet, consult your health provider. This is especially important if you are considering following new treatment recommendations.

Great Uses of the Internet for Getting Health Resources

So now that you know what health information to trust, you can use these tips to find sites that provide information specific to your health condition such as the National Library of Medicine, the Mayo Clinic, or foundations that are specific to the condition you have. The Internet is also great for finding resources to help you cope with the condition you have, such as practitioners considered experts in their field or others with your condition who can provide support. ClinicalTrials.gov, a website that identifies research trials for new treatments, can point you to the doctors conducting those trials, who are often the ones most knowledgeable about that illness. Finding support groups or others with your condition is also made easy with web research. In addition to condition-specific foundations like the Alzheimer's Foundation for caregiver support groups or the American Diabetes Association for diabetes classes, there are a number of online support groups with chat rooms, message boards, and member blogs. While it is best not to take treatment recommendations from these sites, you can get great information on people's experiences with treatment side effects, unusual symptoms, finding practitioners/ hospitals, or just the comfort of knowing that you are not alone in your journey.

Build a Support Network

A support network refers to those individuals in your life whom you can count on when going through a challenging time. They can provide the social, mental, and spiritual support you need. The network may include neighbors, coworkers, family, friends, a religious leader, or fellow worshippers. You may even consider extending your network with the services of a counselor, life coach, or health advocate. Another excellent option for support is the community of individuals dealing your same illness. Others who are going through a similar health challenge can provide practical information based on their experiences. They may also offer emotional support, having been where you are. Even people with a healthy network of family and friends can benefit from the community of others with their illness, because oftentimes, others who have not walked in your shoes don't get it. Finding this community may not be as challenging as you think. One patient, when she found that she had lupus, went immediately to Facebook and found others with the condition from whose experience she could draw. In addition to social networking sites, your doctor, specialist, or local hospital are also great reference sources, especially since many support groups meet at local hospitals. Some health-care providers even have group treatment sessions where several individuals with the same condition agree to have checkups together. They share only what they want to in a group setting, and in addition to providing support to each other, this option can be less expensive. Foundations specific to certain illness, like the America Heart Association, are also treasure troves for finding condition-specific resources, including support groups. And finally, conducting Internet searches can reveal websites where you can share your story and gain support from others.

Regardless of who is in your network, having a network is critical to coping with an illness. Here are some important reasons why: First, social networks give you a health advantage. Studies show that social isolation can be as bad for your health as smoking cigarettes and worse than lack of exercise and being obese. People without strong social connections tend to have higher rates of illness, infection, mental decline, and even death. On the flip side, multiple research studies have shown that stress levels – as measured by stress hormones, blood pressure, and heart rate – are lower in people who have close social support. Brain imaging of people in stressful situations differs between those who are alone versus those who have social support. And the immune systems of people with friends function more effectively, as seen in studies where people with friends stayed healthy more often after exposure to the cold virus compared with those with low social support.

The second reason for a support network is purely practical. At some point, if your illness or treatments for it leave you weak or just take up too much time, you may need a helping hand to ensure your basic needs or daily obligations are met. Family and friends are who we depend on for hands-on support when we are sick – from help doing laundry to making meals and keeping up with medications, appointments, and insurance forms.

Finally – and this is of the highest priority – it is crucial to have a support network to help with advocacy. In the chapters "Relating to Your Doctor" and "Your Hospital Stay – Thriving Through It and Beyond," we will see the key role of an advocate in making sure that your treatment plan suits your individual needs. The only way to be successful in this effort is to have someone who plays the role of your advocate, representing your wishes, making sure you understand all that is happening to you, and ensuring you are benefitting from the care you are getting. When you are well, it is easy to play this role for yourself. But when in pain, nauseated, losing concentration because of medication side effects, or just plain tired, you will miss crucial information. Studies estimate that three of four individuals discharged from an emergency department do not understand either the diagnosis given or their discharge instructions. A good advocate who pays attention to details is not afraid to ask questions until they understand and confidently represent your interests in any situation. If no one in your circle has these skills, you may need to hire someone if you have the resources. It is good to have conversations with your advocate in advance and along the way so they know how you feel about topics like aggressive treatments, what you want done in case your heart stops, you are in a coma, or you cannot breathe on your own. In this way, they can represent your wishes and concerns if necessary. Officially appointing someone as your medical power of attorney will allow that individual to represent your wishes to a doctor or hospital in the event you are not able. Writing those wishes down on paper in a document called "Advanced Directives" will give your medical power of attorney the added confidence that they are representing your true wishes.

Do a Mental Health Check

One of the very first patients I saw as a student in medical school was a young mother hospitalized for shortness of breath. She found out on that admission that she had AIDS and PCP, the pneumonia that develops when your immune system is weak. Despite her severe illness, her main concern was that her husband and young son not find out she had AIDS. On hospital day 3, they found out anyway because she was transferred to the AIDS ward of the hospital. She was crushed when she realized they knew. Although she had started improving, her condition worsened almost overnight, and she died within the next twenty-four hours.

As you think about a shift in perspective, you must to consider your state of mind. If you have a physical health condition, numerous studies have shown that it will be more severe if you are also anxious or depressed. Although not as dramatic as the young mother who had AIDS, anxiety and depression negatively affect many illnesses such as arthritis, asthma, cancer, diabetes, heart failure, obesity, and even back pain. Depression can even result from certain illnesses such as stroke, dementia, heart disease, or brain injury.

For many people, feelings of anxiety and depression can be the natural reaction to a new diagnosis. This response relates to thinking of ourselves as being in great health to suddenly thinking of ourselves as ill or even facing our own mortality. While feelings of despair and sadness are entirely understandable, staying in a place of depression long term stands in the way of your body's ability to cope with your illness and makes your experience of that illness even worse. It also makes it much less likely that you will take care of yourself in an empowered way, a way that will support improvement of your health. For example, research has shown that anxious or depressed persons with diabetes were three times less likely to care properly for themselves compared with people who did not have anxiety and depression.

So for those with a diagnosed illness, one of the most important things you can do for yourself, or if you are a caregiver, for your loved one, is to know the warning signs of depression. Identifying depression is the first step to getting help for it since it is as real an illness as cancer or heart disease. The questions in table 1 are included to help you reflect on your situation or that of someone close to you. It can help identify symptoms that are common in people who are depressed. If you answer yes, you should consider talking to a health professional. If you think that you or someone you know is depressed, it is important to get help.

Table 1:
For the last 2 weeks, have you
 1. felt down, sad, or miserable most of the time?
 2. lost interest or pleasure in most or all of your usual activities?

Other symptoms of depression can include the following: unexpected weight loss or gain (not associated with dieting), problems sleeping, slow movements, a loss of energy or unexplained fatigue, poor appetite, feeling worthless or guilty, problems focusing or concentrating, feeling irritated, frustrated, overwhelmed or indecisive, or having thoughts of death.

Talking with your doctor is a good first step. Because depression can be a symptom of other conditions, he or she may request tests to ensure this is not the case. For treatment, many different options exist. Treatment for depression may include participating in a support group of other persons with your condition, counseling, exercise, light therapy, magnet therapy, or medication. Other well-researched methods that improve symptoms of depression are ones for which you need no prescription. The first includes volunteering or being of service in your community. Science is actually providing evidence for the Biblical adage "it's better to give than receive." Studies show that volunteering can not only help us live longer, recover from illness faster, and prevent diseases, but also help us to experience lower rates of anxiety and depression.

Volunteering and choosing to give to others actually stimulates brain activity associated with feelings of pleasure and reward. Those feelings of pleasure outweigh the symptoms of depression, leading to a greater sense of well-being.

The other way to address depression and anxiety is finding meaning in life through spiritual practice. Spirituality is often defined in terms of meaning and purpose in life, illness, death, and other challenging experiences. When defined in this way, spirituality has been shown to be strongly protective against depression. People receiving treatment for depression often rate their spirituality as one of the most important parts of their recovery.

Takeaway Checklist

Starting with an empowered attitude can make all the difference in your health and the health care you get. To that end, here is your checklist to remind yourself of the steps in that process:

- ☐ Think of yourself as a partner in your care, one with the necessary knowledge and tools to get the best care.
- ☐ You are experiencing an illness – it does not define you.
- ☐ Use the Internet wisely to educate yourself about your condition.
- ☐ Build a support network for emotional support, practical help for your daily activities, and advocacy when you interact with doctors and other health-care personnel.
- ☐ Tune into your mental health and do not hesitate to get help to remove any barriers to effectively caring for yourself.

How Did I Get Here? Common Factors in Dis-Ease – Stress, Inflammation, Genetics, and Lifestyle

Pain (any pain – emotional, physical, mental) has a message. The information it has about our life can be remarkably specific, but it usually falls into one of two categories: "We would be more alive if we did more of this," and, "Life would be lovelier if we did less of that." Once we get the pain's message, and follow its advice, the pain goes away. . . . The more severe the pain or illness, the more severe will be the necessary changes. These may involve breaking bad habits, or acquiring some new and better ones.

– Peter McWilliams, *Life 101*

I have a dear friend who is a true type-A personality, which has helped her to be excellent at her profession. She is a high-energy, always-anxiously-thinking-about-what-she-needs-to-do-next, on-the-go type of person. Her job is stressful, requiring her to have an unusual schedule, staying up twenty-four to thirty-six hours at a time, once or twice a week. In the past five years, she has developed severe heartburn and high blood pressure. I actually did a series of acupuncture treatments on her when she was first getting really severe heartburn symptoms. It relieved the pain, even allowing her to drink wine again without discomfort. The relief lasted for several months but then came right back. Today she is now on Pepcid daily for heartburn; and her doctor plans to start her on medications if her blood pressure readings do not go down in the next three months. Despite the warnings that her body is giving her, she has not yet done anything to address the underlying problem – the level of stress and anxiety in her life.

A NOTHER PART OF becoming empowered to care for yourself is understanding "what is this disease I have" or "how did I end up with this." In many instances, understanding the illness and the reasons you may have it is part of the process of being clear about what role you can play in improving your health. Taking the time to stop and understand what is happening, how you got here, and what changes are required is going from being a passive observer to an active participant in your healing.

While it is too exhaustive to go into the specifics of each and every condition and there are excellent illness-specific resources widely available, it is useful to understand that many diseases share common causes. Knowing these common causes empowers you to address them by making choices that will result in reclaiming better health.

Genes

So what does determine disease? Let's start at the beginning – our genes. The seeds for all health and disease lie in our genes. Genes determine not only our physical makeup but also heavily influence our emotional responses, habits, and predispositions. Our physical makeup can protect us from and, at the same time, make us vulnerable to, certain conditions. However, the degree to which genes determine illness varies greatly. It can be just slightly, like being vulnerable to the common cold virus, to a lot, such as having certain kinds of diseases that run in families, like cancers, sickle cell disease, or birth defects.

All other illness lies somewhere in the middle – diseases that are influenced, both by our genes and also by the lifestyle choices we make, our environment, and our emotional makeup. For example, some people, no matter how much they eat, will never become obese. Others (the majority, unfortunately) are woefully sensitive to what they eat – "a minute on the lips, forever on the hips" – and develop obesity and other related illnesses. The genetic makeup of each of these groups determines whether they manifest obesity or not. For the group that does have the predisposition, it is the choices that they make which cause the expression of this disease. These choices usually are related to what they eat, how they manage stress, and how active they are. In the next section, we will see why these kinds of choices are so important in determining our health.

Chronic Inflammation – Where Stress, Diet, and Lifestyle Meet

Outside of genes, there are several factors that determine if, when, and how severely disease manifests. Doctors are just now beginning to understand that there is a common thread that weaves together stress, nutrition, and lifestyle into a common pathway that leads to many diseases. This common thread is called chronic inflammation. The diseases that are being linked to chronic inflammation are numerous and account for the top reasons for illness in our society. They include heart disease, stroke, brain degenerative diseases like Alzheimer's and Parkinson's disease, type 2 diabetes, obesity, asthma, certain cancer, lupus, fibromyalgias, thyroid diseases like Hashimoto's and Graves' disease, ulcerative colitis, Crohn's disease multiple sclerosis, and rheumatoid arthritis. This is because chronic inflammation can affect every part of the body from the lining of the blood vessels, as in heart disease and stroke, to the pancreas in diabetes, to the muscles and joints in rheumatoid arthritis or fibromyalgia. Here is how it works and why knowing something about what causes it can allow you to influence your own health.

Normally, when the body is at immediate risk from any threat – a muscle strain, exposure to a foreign chemical or virus, or even the development of a cancer cell – it has a tool for defense and repair called the immune system. The body, in its infinite intelligence, sends special cells from the immune system to the area to take care of the problem. The body knows to send these immune cells because any area in trouble signals for help using special "chemical messengers." The entire process of the immune system responding is called inflammation, and the special cells that arrive to save the day are called inflammatory cells. When the job is done, like destroying a cancer cell, the body turns off the chemical messengers that attracted the inflammatory cells, cleans up the scene, and everybody goes home. This process, as you can imagine, happens hundreds of times a day since our bodies are constantly exposed to potential threats.

For reasons that are still not fully understood, there are occasions where this inflammatory process does not stop. The special chemical signals that normally turn off the inflammatory process are never released. As a result, the body continues to send inflammatory cells to disarm the threat even if the problem was already taken care of. This state is called chronic inflammation. There are now blood tests for chronic inflammation that look for high levels of the chemical messengers involved in the inflammation process. For example, doctors are now using C-Reactive Protein or CRP, one of these inflammation chemical messengers, to assess the risk for coronary artery disease, the type of blood vessel disease that can lead to heart attacks.

The location in our body that chronic inflammation shows up is heavily influenced by our genetic makeup and our environmental exposures. If it shows up, when it shows up, and how sick it makes us can depend to a large degree on factors we can influence. These factors include how we respond to the stressors in our life, what we eat, and our weight. Let's look at each of these separately.

Stress: When we become stressed due to life's challenges – pressures at work, financial strain, family arguments – our body switches into high alert, fight-or-flight mode. Because the body thinks it is in danger, it produces alert chemicals that trigger the immune system to turn on. Normally, these alert chemicals would only be produced in short bursts, such as when we are in actual physical danger, and quick action is needed. In today's modern society, where stressors abound, many of us are constantly stressed. As such, we are continuously sending signals for our immune system to stay in an on mode.

Nutrition: What we do eat, or lack in our diet, can also worsen chronic inflammation. Several of the chemical signals and processes the immune system uses to control inflammation require nutrients found in certain foods. If our diet does not have enough of these critical components, like zinc or omega-3 fatty acids, our body will not have the building blocks needed to make the immune system function properly. On the other hand, eating a diet that has substances that irritate our systems also keeps our system in defense mode because the body is constantly trying to neutralize these substances and get them eliminated. Examples of these substances include trans fats, pesticides, and food dyes.

Weight: Obesity fuels many diseases related to chronic inflammation, including arthritis, sleep apnea, heartburn, stroke, heart disease, and high blood pressure. But is obesity itself related to chronic inflammation? The resounding answer from the latest research is yes. Fat plays a vital role in inflammation that we never suspected. So-called apple-shaped people have fat not only visible in their midsection but also inside the body, around the organs where you cannot see it. This hidden fat, called visceral fat, is not just a storage location for extra calories; it releases numerous chemical messengers that promote chronic inflammation all over the body. These fat chemical messengers even affect how hormones like insulin, growth hormone, and sex hormones work in our bodies. This is the reason why those who are apple-shaped have higher rates of diabetes, low sex drive, infertility, in addition to heart disease, stroke, and arthritis. And these effects increase with increasing weight. The risk of diabetes, for example, increases by 9 percent for each kilogram (about every 2 lbs) your weight increases, starting at a BMI of 22. When you get to a BMI over 35, the risk is 40 times higher than those at a normal BMI of 18.5-25. On the flip side, studies are showing that

BMI stands for body mass index and gives an estimate of what you should weigh for your height. To calculate your BMI use weight in kilograms divided by height in meters squared (weight (kg) / [height (m)]²) or go to a BMI calculator website like www.BMIcalculator.com

diet-induced weight loss decreases concentrations of chemical messengers of inflammation like CRP. The bottom line with obesity is that it is a major contributor to many health conditions through its link with chronic inflammation.

There are lifestyle factors which lead to chronic inflammation that when addressed will affect our health and longevity, likelihood of disease, and ability to recover from it. In the next chapter, we will see what we can do to influence the amount of chronic inflammation in our bodies and thus affect how our body can stay well or better function when we are faced with a health challenge.

Takeaway Checklist

☐ Our genes contain the seeds for all health and disease, but the degree to which they manifest is determined by our environment and lifestyle choices.

☐ Stress, our environment, and nutrition all act together to influence our health through chronic inflammation.

☐ Chronic inflammation can lead to the development of multiple conditions.

☐ There are actions we can take to lessen the effects of chronic inflammation on our health.

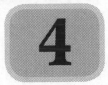

What You Can Do for Yourself

It is much more important to know what sort of a patient has a disease than what sort of a disease a patient has.

– William Osler

I have a friend who is one of the strongest, most resilient people I know. Never a smoker, she had been coughing intermittently for months but thought it was allergies. After finally getting a chest X-ray, she was unfortunately diagnosed with breast cancer that had metastasized or travelled to her lungs. She was in her late thirties when she was diagnosed. The cancer was in an advanced stage which had a very poor prognosis. She had to have surgery and chemotherapy. She was determined, though, that she would maximize her body's ability to heal. To that end, she overhauled her life. She cut out added sugar, alcohol, and meat while upping her intake of vegetables, both raw and cooked, nuts, beans, and fruit. She also started meditating daily and used acupuncture to help get through chemotherapy. Four years later, she is still living and fully participating in life. She still gets regular checkups. However, she has more than beat the odds, not just surviving, but thriving more than three years after she was expected to live.

S O WE HAVE covered the common factors that contribute to illness. And if we stopped here, the picture would look pretty grim. However, it is far from grim because of the many options available to you to minimize the effects of chronic inflammation and the worsening of disease. We are going to dive into what these options are to equip you to be an active partner in your health care and well-being.

Self-Health Actions

For many people with a newly diagnosed condition, it may feel like a sudden change of going from feeling healthy to being ill. However, developing a chronic disease is more like a rock getting worn away by water. It is the daily, almost undetectable changes in your body, like the slow buildup to chronic inflammation, that gradually result in illness. Many people's understanding of being healthy is not having a diagnosed disease or never having been in the hospital. Health actually comes from the Old English word *hale*, meaning "wholeness" and really means that there is wholeness and connection in all levels of our being – body, mind, and soul. This is even reflected in the World Health Organization definition of health as "the state of complete physical, mental, and social well-being and not merely the absence of disease or infirmity."

Because our bodies can absorb a lot of mistreatment over the years, we can, and do, ignore subtle warning signs of ill health and keep trudging along. Chronic inflammation that leads to disease is what happens after a long time of repeating behaviors that we assume will not affect us because we have not felt, or sometimes ignored, the symptoms. It is like starting off on a trip with a full tank of gas. The gas gage is there to let you know when you need to refuel, but unless you pay attention to it, there is no sign that the car is running out of gas until it actually does. Our body is similar in that it will function on all the reserve it has until it runs out. Unless you pay attention to your gages, you will seem to all of a sudden run out of gas, in other words, develop a chronic disease. Health is a state we have to consciously and actively monitor and maintain through the choices that we make. The good news is that even if we do find ourselves in the role of patient, it is rarely too late to make the changes in our lives that can ultimately affect the outcome of our health. The body has amazing powers of recovery, and along with our chosen health-care provider, many options may exist for enabling this self-recovery system to kick in.

Here are some startling statistics about what our body can do. Up to one hundred thousand cancer cells develop in our bodies every day, and if all goes well, which it usually does, they are destroyed, and we never know about them. Each cell in our body has to withstand being bombarded by ten thousand free radicals every second. The heart rebuilds all sixty billion cells it has every seven months, and about two million new red blood cells are released into circulation every second. A healthy immune system that is not bogged down by chronic inflammation is key to helping all these tasks go smoothly. Every choice we make about our health has an impact on how well this dynamic self-recovery system operates.

Given that we are always exposed to irritants and there is nothing we can do about our genes, the best insurance policy for health is to maximize our body's ability to rebound from daily insult. So how do we do this? While there are multiple health supplements, eating programs, and ways of living, I have included below the top five doable self-health actions I think most influence our health throughout our lives and minimize the development of chronic inflammation. For many individuals, these recommendations may represent a radical change from what you are used to or what you think your present lifestyle will allow. However, it is important to realize how Albert Einstein's advice "The significant problems we face cannot be solved at the same level of thinking which created them" definitely applies to our health. The same behaviors, attitudes, and lifestyle choices that contribute to your present state of health, or lack thereof, require adjustment and new thinking if we are to positively affect our health.

Nutrition – Eat Strategically

"Strategic eating" means including those things in your diet that are the building blocks your cells need to thrive, substituting them for the things that are toxic. Vegetables and fruit provide the vitamins and minerals that our bodies need to make our cells work properly, flush toxins, and eliminate natural waste products at the cellular level. The key ingredients that allow our bodies to manufacture the signaling chemicals to turn off chronic inflammation come straight from fruits and vegetables. They create the right chemical balance that allows cells to be happiest and most efficient in carrying out their jobs. They promote the creation of more healthy cells, instead of cancer cells, to replace the cells that die. Eating a plant-based diet will help create this ideal environment needed to repair damage. Other actions that support that optimal environment include:

- Eating single ingredient foods – this means eat only foods that have one ingredient – i.e. eggs, vegetables, fruit, brown rice, sweet potatoes, water, lean meat, and fish. By sticking to this as much as possible, you automatically will eliminate processed foods, sugary beverages, and foods with added salt and sugar.
- Drinking eight ounces of fresh vegetable juice daily – juicing is a great way to ensure the body gets adequate amounts of vegetables every day without having to eat them all.

- Including healthy fats – avocado, coconut, olive oil, fatty fish – in your diet daily. You can even add coconut oil to your daily vegetable juice to make sure you get this in. Healthy fats actually have components needed for the repair of cells and are the building blocks of the brain.

- Avoiding foods in your diet that are potential irritants such as wheat and soy products. One way to figure out if they are irritants for you is to eliminate them altogether for two weeks and then gradually add them back into your diet. If you add them back in and then get the common signs of bodily irritation – bloating, headaches, irritability/mood changes, constipation or diarrhea, fatigue – you know they are not for you. Irritant foods promote chronic inflammation in the body, so avoiding them is key for improving health.

There are numerous stories describing the beneficial effects of juicing and raw diets on changing the course of illness. One close to me is my seventy-eight-year-old father-in-law. Plagued for years with the chronic health challenges of diabetes, high blood pressure, and hardening of the arteries, he started to juice just this year. By adding freshly made vegetable-based juices to his diet, he lost twelve pounds in two months. He gained the energy to start walking again, and his doctor is starting to lessen the doses of the medicines he takes. He is an inspiration to me and proves it is never too late to make change!

Get Ten to Fifteen Minutes of Sunlight Daily

Did you know research suggests that not getting enough direct sunlight, specifically ultraviolet (UVB) rays, significantly increases our chances of cancer? Natural UVB rays from sunlight convert cholesterol in our bare skin to vitamin D. Our livers and kidneys then do their magic and turn vitamin D into a hormone, calcitriol, that goes to all the cells throughout our bodies. If we were to expose at least 20 percent of our skin to sunlight all year round for up to ten minutes a day without any SPF, then we would ensure adequate amounts of vitamin D. The best sun exposure during summer is about ten minutes of morning sun before 9:00 a.m. or late afternoon after 5:00 p.m. In the winter, about twenty minutes is needed. UVB rays are the only ones that actually trigger the vitamin D in our body, so solariums or sun tan beds will only be helpful if they radiate ultraviolet rays.

Obstacles to vitamin D conversion are all the enemies of direct sunlight – northern latitude locations, cloudy atmospheres, darker seasons, and pollution. Additionally, melanin acts as a light filter, so individuals with more melanin in their skin (darker skin) need more time to absorb enough sunlight for vitamin D synthesis. For people with very fair skin, a short burst of sunshine on their skin is enough to get vitamin D conversion going. For everyone, it is still important to monitor your time in the sun, as too much UVB is not necessarily a good thing. If planning to stay out longer, using natural, chemical-free SPF 15 + sunscreen found in health food stores can protect for your skin. Because of the role of the liver and kidney in the vitamin D production, people with liver or kidney disease require more vitamin D either from direct sunlight or oral intake.

So why is getting Vitamin D so crucial? It has been long known that vitamin D helps us absorb calcium and maintain healthy strong bones and teeth. Without it, bones can become thin, brittle, soft, or misshapen, leading to rickets in children and osteoporosis in adults. In addition, vitamin D is important in determining proper cell functioning which explains why recent Vitamin D research shows its relationship to breast, colon, and skin cancer. The research study done at Creighton University Medical School in Nebraska showed that those participants receiving calcium and vitamin D supplements showed at least 60 percent decrease in cancers. Insufficient vitamin D has also been associated with other conditions including Alzheimer's, allergies, autoimmune disorders, like multiple sclerosis and rheumatoid arthritis, depression, both type 1 and 2 diabetes, heart disease, high blood pressure, infertility, sexual dysfunction, learning and behavior disorders, obesity, osteopenia, osteoporosis, Parkinson's disease, PMS, and psoriasis.

As an alternative to sunlight, the required daily amount of Vitamin D3 is 400 International Units (IU) taken orally. It is imperative to have a simple blood test from your doctor to check your current levels of vitamin D before considering any supplementation. This will help to avoid the effect of oversupplementing, which can be harmful to bones and other tissues. After you start Vitamin D supplements, get your levels rechecked four months later to see if you have corrected the deficiency. Foods that contain Vitamin D3 and the amounts are

* 1 tablespoon cod liver oil – 1,360 IU
* 100gr (3.5 oz) salmon, cooked – 360 IU
* 100gr (3.5 oz) mackerel, cooked – 345 IU
* 100gr (3.5 oz) sardines, canned in oil, drained – 270 IU
* 250ml (8 fl oz or 1 cup) milk, nonfat, reduced fat, and whole, vitamin D fortified – 98 IU
* 1 whole egg, soft boiled (vitamin D is present in the yolk) – 25 IU

Sleep Well

Sleep experts recommend at least seven to eight hours of sleep a night for most adults. For kids under one, the minimum is fourteen hours; one- to three-year-olds need at least twelve hours; three- to twelve-year-olds need at least nine to ten hours, and twelve to eighteen about eight to nine hours. But no matter our age, most of us average less than what we need. The National Sleep Foundation has shown that adults typically get less than seven hours a night during the work week and 90 percent of American parents erroneously think that their child is getting enough sleep. Half of all adolescents get less than seven hours of sleep on weeknights. By the time they are seniors in high school, according to studies by the University of Kentucky, they average only slightly more than 6.5 hours of sleep a night. Only 5 percent of high school seniors average eight hours. It has been documented in a handful of major studies that children, from elementary school through high school, get about an hour less sleep each night than they did 30 years ago, and even kindergartners get 30 minutes less a night than they used to.

Where it may not seem like a big deal to miss some hours of sleep, the consequences of being sleep deprived may seem surprising. Undersleeping can lead to:

- Getting sick more often: Being rested keeps our immune systems in tune to be able to prevent infections. When we miss sleep, we have fewer and weaker T-cells, the main fighter cells of our immune system. Hence, we are more likely to get infections like colds and flu.

- Higher likelihood of dying: Adults who sleep less than six hours a night compared to those who get more than seven hours nightly are more likely to die from all causes, including heart attacks.

- Weight gain and type 2 diabetes: Sleep deprivation promotes weight gain and type 2 diabetes in similar ways. First of all, when our body is not rested, it perceives that it is under stress. It then releases the stress hormones, cortisol and insulin. Both high insulin and high cortisol level encourage the buildup of body fat. Also, with higher levels of insulin hanging around, the body becomes less sensitive to its effects, leading to type 2 diabetes. Sleep deprivation can also promote weight gain by affecting our behavior. Because of flagging energy during the day, sleep-deprived people will turn to calorie-dense foods for an energy burst. However, the extra calories are not needed by the body and are therefore stored as body fat. Sleep-deprived people are often too tired to exercise, or they work out less intensely than usual.

- Short stature: In children, a chronic lack of sleep can lead to stunting of growth because growth hormone is released when we sleep.

- Brain power: For adults, undersleeping can result in lack of focus and poor concentration. The effects of undersleeping are even more profound in children. This is because children's brains are still developing until age twenty-five, and much of that development happens during sleep. Hyperactivity, poor academic performance, and lack of emotional stability in children are all linked to getting just one less hour of sleep per night on average.

Many people simply cannot fall asleep or have a hard time staying asleep. Especially as we age, sleep becomes more difficult. Sleep hygiene is the practice of making one's environment and body more ready for sleep when the time is right. Even though some of the suggestions seem obvious, many people do not follow them, leading to poor sleep habits.

Personal Habits

- **Be consistent in your bedtime and awakening time.** Your body gets used to falling asleep at a certain time, but only if this time is relatively fixed. A migrating bedtime can confuse the body about when to become sleepy.
- **Avoid extensive napping during the day.** Napping is not a bad thing to do, but for adults, it is best to limit the nap to thirty to forty-five minutes so that the majority of sleep can occur at night.
- **Avoid alcohol, caffeine, and heavy or sugary foods four to six hours before bedtime.** When the sleep-inducing effects of alcohol wear off in few hours, there is a stimulant or wake-up effect. It can often be difficult to fall back to sleep after this. Sugary foods and caffeinated beverages such as coffee, tea, colas, and other caffeinated sodas and chocolate can all have a stimulant effect. Both alcohol and caffeine can increase nighttime urination, leading to more frequent awakening. Heavy or spicy foods can lead to heartburn, especially worse when lying down, which can affect your ability to fall and stay asleep.

- **Exercise regularly.** Regular exercise can help deepen sleep. The conventional wisdom of not exercising close to bedtime is changing based on the 2013 *Sleep in America®* poll, which found that exercise done anytime, even close to bedtime, is effective at improving sleep quality.

Your Sleeping Environment

- **Make your bedding and bedroom comfy**. Poor mattress quality or an uncomfortable pillow can all impede a good night's sleep, and both should be changed on a regular basis. Cooler temperature and good ventilation promote sleep while a too cold, too hot, or too stuffy room can keep you awake.

- **Block out all distracting noise, and eliminate as much light as possible.** For safety purposes, especially with children or older adults, a night light may provide just enough light not to disturb sleep but allow for safely getting out of bed if needed.

- **Reserve the bed for pleasurable activities like sleep and sex.** Don't use the bed as an office or workroom. Let your body know that the bed is associated with sleeping and is a stress-free environment.

Getting Ready For Bed

- **Try a light snack before bed.** Many people cannot go to sleep hungry. A light snack on foods high in the amino acid tryptophan – spinach, seaweed, turkey, tofu, egg whites, warm milk – can help you fall asleep.

- **Relax at bedtime.** Incorporate practices that can help you relax such as yoga, prayer, and deep breathing to help to relieve anxiety and allow muscle tension to go away. Bedtime rituals like a warm bath or a few minutes of reading can also serve as relaxation techniques.

- **Avoid television, cell phone, computer, and video game at bedtime**. Many people try to sleep with the television on in their room. Television is a very engaging medium that tends to keep people up. As a result, watching television before bedtime or in the middle of the night does not promote relaxation and sleep. Violent content can even promote bad dreams. For people with chronic problems sleeping, it is a good idea for the television not to be in the bedroom. Other overstimulating media for children and teens include video games, computers, and cell phones and prevent relaxation at bedtime. For those who feel they need some sound to sleep, talk radio or soothing music is an alternative since they are less engaging media.

Getting Up in the Middle of the Night

If you wake up during the night for various reasons and cannot get back to sleep within twenty minutes, remaining in the bed trying to fall asleep can be counterproductive. Doing this tends to make you watch the clock and just worry about the sleep you are not getting. Instead, if you switch to a calming pastime like reading, light snacking, or meditation, you will more likely slip back into dreamland. Challenging or engaging activities like office work, housework, or strenuous exercise will be counterproductive and result in getting you revved up.

Following these sleep suggestions faithfully will help the majority of children and adults with sleep problems. However, for those individuals who continue to have problems even after these measures, other conditions need to be considered. This is the time to consult a health-care professional to help determine the problem and the best treatment. Medications can cause sleeplessness as a side effect and a review of all medications should be done with adjustments made if possible. Underlying medical conditions that cause sleeplessness, like sleep apnea or restless leg syndrome, should be investigated. Only if all options are exhausted should a prescribed sleep aide be tried since these products vary in safety and effectiveness and are rarely meant for more than short-term use. The ultimate goal is being able to fall asleep naturally.

Drink!

No, not alcohol, but other liquids, especially water. Our bodies are made up of, on average, 70 percent water. Our bodies are always using up water and so are in constant need of fluid replenishment. The numbers tell the story. Breathing alone gets rid of two to four cups of water each day. Sweating accounts for another two cups of water, and this does not include exercise-induced perspiration. And every trip to the bathroom to urinate is about a cup of water. So with just normal living, you got through at least eight cups a day. And we have not even touched on extra water loss that happens when we are sick – vomiting, diarrhea, runny nose, cough – or losses associated with diuretics like caffeine or medications for high blood pressure.

Unless we replace these losses, dehydration is the result. The medical definition of dehydration is losing 10 percent or more of your body weight in fluids. However, it takes a lot less than that to start to feel subtle symptoms that we rarely associate with not being adequately hydrated. As little as 2 percent of your body weight in water loss can affect mood and cause headaches, body aches, sleepiness, fatigue, lack of focus, and dull thinking abilities. Two percent for a standard 170-pound individual is only about 6 cups. Adequate water intake can also help headaches and sore muscles by improving circulation and should be the first remedy before pain medicines for these common ailments. In addition, adequate water consumption can help lessen the chance of kidney stones, keep joints lubricated, prevent and lessen the severity of colds and flu, and help prevent constipation.

How do you know how much fluid to drink daily? Unless a real effort is made to keep up with losses, it is easy to not get enough fluid daily. Here are three ways to go about it. You can pick the one that works best for you:

- **Replacement approach.** Between urine, breath, sweat, and bowel movements, we lose close to 2.5 liters of water a day. Food usually accounts for 20 percent of your fluid intake, so drinking 2 liters of water or other beverages a day (a little more than 8 cups), along with your normal diet takes care of lost fluids. An easy way to remember this is the 8 x 8 rule – drinking eight 8-ounce glasses of water/fluids a day (about 1.9 liters).
- **Dietary recommendations.** The Institute of Medicine recommends that men consume 3 liters (about 13 cups) of total beverages a day and women consume 2.2 liters (about 9 cups) of total beverages a day.
- **Follow your body.** If all else fails, drink enough water to quench your thirst and produce a colorless to slightly yellow urine. Thirst is sometimes mistaken as hunger, so a good strategy is to first drink liquids, preferably water, when you think you are hungry.

Special fluid considerations: Another water-related pitfall is not accounting for the increased fluids needed when consuming beverages that contain caffeine like teas, coffee, and certain sodas, or alcohol. Caffeine and alcohol of any kind are diuretics, so even though you take in fluid while consuming them, you actually need to increase your total fluid intake to compensate. The common hangover is really dehydration and actually can be avoided by drinking enough water before going to bed or upon rising the next day.

For individuals with diabetes, adequate water intake is essential because high blood sugars can worsen dehydration, and drinking water helps to keep blood sugar regulated. The following tips are helpful for people with diabetes, but everyone can benefit from them:

- Drink a glass of water with each meal and between each meal.
- Take water breaks instead of coffee or tea breaks.
- Substitute sparkling water for alcoholic drinks at social gatherings.

There are certain diseases like heart failure or kidney disease in which water is not being handled properly by your body. Intake must be individually determined in consultation with your doctor. Be sure to consult with your doctor to determine the ideal water intake for you if you have one of these conditions.

Develop Your Healthy Way of Dealing with Stress

When I was seven years old, I was really into Archie comic books. For whatever reason, I still remember a phrase I read way back then that stuck with me: "Don't be a thermometer, be a thermostat." As I got older and finally knew what a thermostat was, it really made sense. Rather than react to a stressful situation by having our temperature rise to match the situation, like a thermometer does, maintain an even temperature no matter what is going on, like a thermostat. Being a thermometer means we are letting our perception of the situation control us and our response. Being a thermostat means maintaining an inner calm no matter what is going on around us. This can even influence the situation to be less stressful. In order to be able to be a thermostat and not a thermometer, it takes working out our own individual way of maintaining our inner equilibrium. It also turns out that there are tremendous health benefits to being a thermostat. Let us look into how this can be possible.

Is "Stress" Really So Bad?

Let us first talk about why having stressors in our life is beneficial. The challenges in our life, also known as stressors, help us to grow to adapt to new situations. Because the world is constantly changing, if we do not change with it, we would be "stuck in a rut" and would not last very long. Stressors motivate us to problem solve and accomplish and learn new skills to adapt to ever changing situations.

So why does stress have such a bad rap? Because stressors and stress are two different things. Stressors are only the situations we experience. Stress is our own perception of the situation. We subjectively experience stress when, according to the definition of stress, we think the demands of the situation "exceed the personal and social resources the individual is able to mobilize." In other words, we think a situation is too much for us to manage or is out of our control. However, it rarely is, and our ability to cope is entirely determined by our mind-set. A good example of this is people on a roller coaster ride. For some it is a terrifying experience never to be repeated; others sit carefree at the front of the ride, hands thrown up in the air in glee, and yet others in the middle are bored. Depending on whom you ask, you will get a different answer to "was the roller coaster ride stressful?" The main difference was the perception of each person about the control they felt they had over the event. Many times, we create our own stress because of learned responses and end up being stressed. When this happens on a daily basis, we have chronic stress, which can lead to chronic inflammation and poor health.

The point where the positive effects of having a stressor cross over in to the paralyzing effects of chronic stress varies from person to person. It is important to be sensitive to the early warning signs that suggest you are crossing that point into the danger zone. Such signals differ for each of us and can be so subtle that they are often ignored until it is too late. What do I mean by too late? "Too late" means our bodies start to feel the effects of a constant perception of stress in our daily lives that we have not been effectively managing. For our bodies to be in their best state of health, it is therefore important to (1) know how to repair our bodies from the effects of being chronically stressed, (2) develop good or adaptive ways of dealing with stressors – ways that help us to continue to function well despite stress – and (3) develop techniques to avoid becoming stressed altogether.

Repairing from the Physical Effects of Chronically "Being Stressed"

The first is dealing with chronic inflammation, the physical result of chronically "being stressed" that we discussed previously. Our body goes into crisis mode (becomes sick) from the long-term exposure to chronic stress. We first have to repair from this crisis mode, regardless of the crisis – type 2 diabetes, cancer, back pain, heartburn, or lupus. I call treatments done in crisis "salvage mode". Repairing in salvage mode likely will require one or more of the many different treatments we use when we are sick. It can involve taking medications like insulin, blood pressure pills, or antacids, complementary approaches like acupuncture, homeopathy, physical therapy, massage, or even surgery for extremely advanced illnesses like cancers. It depends upon what is being treated, your preference for the treatment, and the professional advice you receive.

Techniques for Managing Daily Stress – Maintenance Mode

At the same time we are treating crisis mode, we can start to address some of the factors that resulted in us getting to that point. If successful, we may be able to leave crisis mode behind and continue to employ these same strategies to maintain our health gains. I call this maintenance mode. A critical factor that needs to be addressed is how we manage the effects of daily stress in our lives. The good news is that there are a variety of different strategies to effectively manage how we process stress on a day-to-day basis.

The first is to have ways to relax and focus our attention away from our stressors. By practicing these relaxation techniques, the goal is eventually to be able to tune into that state of mind at will. There are techniques for that too. The movements, breathing, and focus used in Yoga, Tai Chi, and Qigong are intended to result in relaxation, concentration, and balance. Although these disciplines are each from different traditions, the effect of each practiced consistently is to strengthen the body and clear the mind. Qigong, over five thousand years old, is considered a branch of Chinese medicine along with acupuncture, massage, and herbs. Tai Chi dates back to the 1600s and is rooted in the internal nonaggressive forms of martial arts. Even though Tai Chi has martial arts roots, most modern Tai Chi has evolved to be used for health. Yoga, originally from India, uses postures to make the body a stronger place for meditation and spiritual development. Studies show that the regular practice of Yoga, at least three times a week, can actually reduce the levels of stress hormones circulating in our system. All three forms of exercise have the potential to reduce and prevent chronic inflammation in the body through regular practice.

Regular aerobic exercise, like dancing, swimming, walking, or biking is useful in removing the by-products of the stress response from our system. Because your body is engaged in the physical activity that your body expects when under stress, regular exercise allows the body to return to a normal state faster and reduce the physical impact of being stressed. It also is an outlet for anger and other toxic emotions. Like Yoga, Tai Chi, and Qigong, aerobic exercise also moves muscles which are chronically tense from stress. Exercise of some sort is the most common and most accessible way to burn off those excess stress hormones that build up. Regular moderate exercise has been shown to have a positive effect on all organs, starting with the nervous system, through improved learning and memory, mood, and protection against brain degeneration such as in Alzheimer's and Parkinson's disease. Cancer of the colon, breast, prostate, endometrium, pancreas, and skin are all more common in inactive individuals, compared to those who exercise. Unlike exercising too long (over 1.5 hours) or too hard, which does not help the immune system, regular, moderate exercise has been shown to reduce the body's inflammation. Moderate exercise, according to the Department of Health and Human Services, is a level of exertion that raises your heart rate to a point where you sweat and feel you are working, yet you can still carry on a conversation.

There are also many non-exercise based forms of relaxation. Because breathing is one of the first bodily responses to change when we experience stress, deep-power breathing is an easily accessible way to relaxation. Other forms of relaxation include developing a hobby that you love in which you can get lost when you do it – knitting, reading, woodworking, gardening, playing a musical instrument.

Whatever practice you do to address stress in your life, do it on a daily basis is the key. The stress reactions we have occur on a daily basis, and it is better to deal with the effects as they occur rather than waiting for them to accumulate.

Living beyond Stress

So we know about repairing the effects of advanced stress in the salvage mode. We have also learned about dealing with stress on a day to day basis after it happens or maintenance mode. The ultimate protection from stress is to have techniques to avoid becoming stressed altogether, what I call living beyond stress. Since being stressed is a learned response, wouldn't it be great if we could unlearn those responses and learn different ones? There are actually tools for doing just that. Hypnosis and cognitive behavioral therapy, described in subsequent chapters, both can help us to reinterpret our being-stressed triggers. In addition, any technique that promotes and reestablishes connection to one's inner self or spirit promotes living beyond the level of stress. Meditation is one such well-studied technique. Daily meditation reestablishes an alpha brain wave state of relaxation, decreases stress hormones in the blood, and produces long-lasting changes in the brain activity in areas involved in attention, working memory, learning, and conscious perception. There is a growing body of scientific research that links meditation to reductions in high blood pressure, reversal of hardening of the arteries known to lead to strokes and heart attacks, and even an extended life span. In addition to heart and blood disease, research shows some benefit in a wide range of conditions such as anxiety, asthma, binge eating, cancer, depression, fatigue, heart disease, high blood pressure, pain management, sleep problems, and substance abuse. In controlled research trials, individuals who meditated had less release of the stress hormone cortisol, indicating a greater improvement in their ability to regulate their response to stress. In addition, the meditators, in contrast to the comparison group who was taught only how to relax, showed lower levels of anxiety, depression, anger, and fatigue. How does meditation do this? Neuroscientists have found that meditators shift their brain activity away from the stress-prone areas in the right frontal cortex of the brain to the calmer left frontal cortex. This mental shift decreases the negative effects of stress, mild depression, and anxiety. It also appears to lessen the activity in the area where the brain processes fear, called the amygdala.

So what kind of meditation works best? Whichever kind works best for you. There are any number of ways to meditate. Silent prayer is one form. Another form often used by beginners is just focusing attention on breathing deeply as you inhale and exhale slowly through your nostrils. You can also expand your practice to concentration meditation, which involves focusing one's attention on the breath, an imagined or real image, ritualized movements (as in Tai Chi, Yoga, or Qigong), or on a sound, word, or phrase that is repeated silently or aloud (mantra). When thoughts or emotions arise, the person gently directs his or her mind back to the original focus of concentration. In the Christian tradition, chanting and saying the rosary are forms of concentration meditation. (A rosary is a string of beads used to keep track of the prayers recited.) Movement meditation may be spontaneous and free form, or it may involve highly structured, choreographed, repetitive patterns, as in the practice of Tai Chi or Qigong. Movement meditation is particularly helpful for those people who find it difficult to remain still.

Regardless of how you do concentration meditation, the purpose is to fully experience the present moment with serenity. The benefit of being fully present is that worries and anxieties fade, and a feeling of peace ensues. It is the feeling of peace that has physical benefits in the body and has been referred to as the relaxation response. In contrast to concentration meditation, yet another technique is mindfulness meditation, which involves becoming aware of the entire field of attention. There is an awareness of all thoughts, feelings, perceptions, or sensations as they arise from moment to moment. Mindfulness meditation is enhanced by the person's ability to quiet the mind and to accept all that they perceive with a sense of composure.

Whatever approach to meditation you choose – concentrating on the sensation of the movement of the breath, silently repeating a mantra, chanting a prayer, visualizing a peaceful and meaningful place, focusing awareness on the center of the body, increasing awareness of all sensory experiences, some hybrid of these or a different one altogether – there are clear benefits to your health. You can essentially reset your brain to start living beyond the negative effects of stress on our bodies. The ultimate goal, regardless of your current state of health, is to lessen the high levels of stress hormones, chronic inflammation, and other factors that wear the body down over time.

Takeaway Checklist

Incorporating self-health actions in your routine can lessen the opportunity for chronic inflammation to form. These self-health actions include:

- ☐ Eat single ingredient foods.
- ☐ Drink eight ounces of vegetable juice a day – find a good book on juicing recipes and talk with your health-care provider about get started.
- ☐ Avoid irritant foods – the most common ones are wheat and soy.
- ☐ Eat healthy fats.
- ☐ Get adequate Vitamin D ideally through at least ten minutes of sunlight a day.

☐ Create the right conditions to get seven to eight hours of sleep a night.

☐ Drink enough water to stay well hydrated and remove waste.

☐ Choose and practice daily ways to manage the effects of stress in your life.

What Health-Care Providers Do You Need on Your Team?

There is no alternative medicine. There is only medicine that works and medicine that doesn't work.

– Richard Dawkins

My mother grew up as the daughter of a country doctor in a small North Carolina town. As the general practitioner (GP) there, he did everything. He took care of all the townspeople, bringing them into this world, caring for them while they were here, and pronouncing them as they left. I never knew him, but based on stories, he did this with empathy and compassion. Because it was a town of only two thousand people, he knew his patients and their families personally, so he provided holistic care. People believed in his treatments. He also accepted payments in chickens, eggs, and rabbits. To this day, my mother cannot understand why she cannot find a doctor to care for her like her dad did for the townspeople, or why referrals to specialists are so commonly done.

A CRUCIAL STEP IN focusing on your health is choosing your professional partner in health. Today, though, getting care has evolved from a simple relationship with a GP. Because of the exponential increase in medical knowledge, it now takes a team approach to bring it all to bear in caring for patients. The health-care team is the collection of professionals you engage to help you manage your health and well-being. There is a huge variety of types of practitioners out there to choose from, so it is important to know what each of them can do for you. The goal of this chapter is to review the various kinds of doctors, both conventional and alternative, and the services they provide, then highlight other nonmedical members of health-care team you will encounter.

Know What Type of Doctor You Are Looking For

Your ideal health professional is really determined by your health concerns, the time you are willing to invest in a treatment plan, and your philosophy of health. Do you need a primary health-care provider (a doctor who will manage your overall care and refer you to specialists when necessary)? Or do you need a specialist in a particular area? A conventional doctor, an alternative practitioner, or one who combines both? Before you decide, become familiar with all the various types of comprehensive health-care practitioners. This is not meant to be an exhaustive list but includes the most visited types of practitioners.

- Allopathic MDs – conventional or western medicine
- Osteopathic physicians
- Naturopaths
- Integrative practitioners
- Chiropractors
- Homeopaths
- Acupuncturists/traditional Chinese medicine
- Ayurvedic Practitioners

So how do you know who to seek out? Not only are there a wide array of health practitioners, but even among conventional western doctors, there are various specialists. This chapter sets the record straight on who does what, and also offers tips, where backed up by research studies, for who is best at what. It also lets you know the philosophy of health of each type of practitioner, so you can see if it aligns with yours. No matter who you choose, though, the best thing you can do is to tell all your health-care providers about other treatments you are getting or considering. Give them a full picture of all you do to manage your health. This will ensure coordinated and safe care.

Allopathic Doctors

What They Do: Allopathy is the big umbrella for the system of conventional western medicine. The term *allopathy* was coined in the nineteenth century and has since come to describe the philosophy of modern medicine based upon understanding the disease and treatments through scientific enquiry and research. It uses *medicines* or *physical interventions* like surgery or physical therapy to treat or suppress *symptoms* or disease processes. These practitioners are known as doctors of medicine and have the initials MD after their names. Within allopathic medicine are specialists based upon their areas of training.

Primary Care

Primary-care doctors are generally the first stop when something ails you, and if your problem is beyond their scope, they will refer you to the right specialist. They also provide preventive care, like helping you lose weight, providing vaccines like the flu shot or screenings, like prostate exams or mammograms. The primary-care doctor for adults is called an internist/ internal medicine doctor, and for children, a pediatrician. Family medicine doctors, previously called generalists, also provide primary care, but for the entire family, regardless if age. In some rural areas, family medicine doctors even deliver babies, although this is becoming much less common.

Women of child-bearing age often use obstetrician-gynecologists (OB-GYNs) as their primary-care physicians since many health concerns in this group are reproductive in nature. OB-GYNs care for women's reproductive health, deliver babies, and perform surgery on the female reproductive system. Geriatricians are primary-care doctors, either family practitioners or internists, who care for older adults and have additional training in problems unique to aging.

Nurse practitioners (NP), although not MDs, provide primary care as well, often in areas where there are shortages of doctors. NPs are advanced nurses with graduate-level education who hold national board certification in an area of specialty and are licensed through the state nursing boards. They see individuals of all ages depending on their specialty (family, pediatrics, geriatrics, etc.) and treat both physical and mental conditions using the same techniques an allopathic physician does. Because they can prescribe medication, practice without physician supervision, and be reimbursed directly by insurance companies, some nurse practitioners have their own practices where they serve as a primary-care provider. Other NPs practice in a team environment with physicians, referring persons with more complex problems for the physician's care.

When you have more than one doctor, it is best to have a primary-care provider who can coordinate the care you are receiving. Many medical errors result from the lack of one health provider who has the overall picture of the various treatments that are being provided to an individual. For example, without one person who has the big picture, a medication can be started by one doctor that counteracts the effects of another treatment from a different doctor. A good primary-care practitioner ensures that all care provided is done in a coordinated fashion, much like a conductor directing orchestra. There are still many challenges to this happening seamlessly. However, with the electronic documentation now being widely adopted and the ability to send information between practitioners, the coordination of care is becoming a reality, so the right hand can know what the left is doing.

Health-care reform has been able to promote the idea of the Patient-Centered Medical Home (PCMH), where primary-care doctors work with teams of other health professionals like nurse practitioners, therapists, health educators, and pharmacists, to make sure that all your needs are met at each visit. Electronic documentation makes sure that each health-care team member knows about each individual's health concerns, diagnoses, allergies, and medications so that no mistakes are made. And most importantly, in the medical home model, doctors are held accountable for whether their patients' health improves or not since part of their pay is actually based on how their patients are doing as a whole. The health-care team members ensure that you, as the health-care consumer, understand and are in agreement with the plan of care and have everything you need to successfully carry it out. Some practices are even adopting patient portals, secure websites where you can be updated on all your medical information, schedule appointments, get medication refills, and receive health education. The PCMH is designed to improve the individual user's experience as a health-care consumer, and it may be helpful to look for a doctor whose practice has switched to this way of improving the quality of care they provide.

Specialist Care

Many internal medicine doctors go on to specialize and even subspecialize in areas related to the major internal organ systems.

These include cardiologists for the heart, pulmonologists for the lungs, gastroenterologists for the intestinal tract, hepatologists for the liver (a subspecialty of gastroenterology), and nephrologists for the kidney. Other internal medicine–based specialists include endocrinologists, whose focus is the endocrine or hormone system, which includes thyroid disease and diabetes; hematologists whose focus is the blood which would include treating sickle cell disease; infectious disease doctors; allergists/immunologists who focus on the immune system; and oncologists who focus on cancer care. These doctors, with rare exception, treat conditions with medications and do not perform surgery.

Which brings us to the other major division within allopathic medicine, the surgery-based disciplines. These include general surgeons who technically can perform surgery anywhere in the body. However, because of the complexity of the human body and advanced surgical techniques, surgeons too have chosen to specialize. General surgeons operate mainly on the abdomen. Thoracic surgeons focus on organs in the chest, such as the heart, lungs, and esophagus. Vascular surgeons operate on blood vessels. Other surgeons include orthopedic or bone surgeons; neurosurgeons, who focus on the brain, spinal cord, and major nerves; plastic surgeons who operate on facial and other surface features of the body and do cosmetic surgery; urologists for the urinary system of both sexes and the male reproductive system; and ear, nose, and throat (ENT) surgeons also called otolaryngologists.

There are other specialists who fall outside the broad division of medicine and surgery. Emergency medicine specialists stabilize individuals in the first few hours of an illness or trauma. Anesthesiologists administer anesthesia before surgical procedures and also subspecialize in pain medicine, the management of chronic pain; dermatologists care for the skin and do skin surgical procedures; obstetrician-gynecologists, who deliver babies and focus on the reproductive health of women; psychiatrists, who specialize in mental health; and physical medicine and rehabilitation doctors, who care for individuals who are recovering from catastrophic illness like strokes, paraplegia, or sports injuries. Radiologists interpret all the various types of pictures taken of the body including CT scans, MRIs, and X-rays, and some subspecialize in interventional radiology, the use of catheter wires to entire hard-to-reach parts of the body as an alternative to surgery. Finally, there are pathologists who use microscopes to examine small sections of the body to diagnose disease and determine ideal treatment, such as in the diagnosis and treatment of certain cancers. Forensic pathologists, seen on TV shows like CSI, figure out the cause of death, a process called an autopsy.

There are also doctors who you will only find in a hospital. Examples include hospitalists, who care for individuals when they are hospitalized, and intensivists/critical care doctors, who care for individuals in the intensive care unit (ICU). Finally, if hospitalized in a teaching hospital, you may also encounter students and doctors who have not yet finished their training. These include medical students in one of their four years; interns, in their first year out of medical school; residents, who have finished medical school and internship, and are taking anywhere from three to seven years to pursue a specialty like internal medicine or surgery; or fellows, who typically have finished residency training and are subspecializing in a discipline like cardiology or vascular surgery.

In addition, there may be further sub-specialization based upon factors like age, like pediatric hematologists, who only care for children with blood diseases; or upon factors such as type of disease or severity of disease such as gynecologic oncologists, who focus on cancers of the female reproductive system; or high-risk obstetricians, who focus on caring for women with high-risk pregnancies.

The following chart (figure 5-1) can help if you are trying to determine what role an MD can play for you.

Figure 5-1 Allopathic Physicians and What They Do

Medicine-based

Generalists	What they do	Examples of common scenarios/conditions treated
Internal Medicine (Internists)	General medicine for adults	Initial evaluation and management of symptoms, annual exams, vaccinations
Family Medicine	General medicine for adults and children – the whole family	Initial evaluation and management of symptoms, annual exams, vaccinations
Pediatricians	General medicine for children	Initial evaluation and management of symptoms, well-child visits, vaccinations
Geriatricians	Care for older adults and focus on problems unique to aging	Poor mobility, arthritis, osteoporosis, dementia

Medical and Pediatric Specialists	What they do	Examples of common conditions treated
Cardiologists	Heart specialists	Heart attacks, heart failure
Pulmonologists	Lung specialists	COPD, asthma, pneumonia
Gastroenterologist	Digestive tract specialists – stomach, intestines, colon, gallbladder, pancreas, liver	Stomach ulcers, pancreatitis, Crohn's disease
Neurologists	Nervous system and brain specialists	Strokes, Parkinson's disease, Alzheimer's Disease
Nephrologist	Kidney specialists	Kidney failure
Endocrinologist	Endocrine system specialists	Thyroid disease, diabetes
Hematologist	Blood disease specialists	Sickle cell disease, thalassemia, leukemia
Oncologist	Cancer specialists	Any cancer including prostate, lung, breast, and colon cancers
Infectious Disease	Contagious disease specialists – illnesses caused by viruses, bacteria, and fungi	HIV, sepsis (overwhelming blood infection), pneumonia, meningitis
Rhuematologist	Movement system specialists – joints, muscles, soft tissues around the joints and bones	Rheumatoid arthritis, lupus, gout
Allergist/ Immunologist	Immune system specialists	Asthma, eczema, allergic reactions to drugs, foods, and insect stings; diseases related to a poorly functioning immune system like HIV
Neonatolgists	Newborn infants generally while in the hospital	Prematurely born infants

Surgery-based

Specialty	What they do	Examples of common scenarios/conditions treated
General Surgery	Can operate on any body part but generally stick with the abdomen since there are so many other specialists	Appendicitis
Orthopedics	Surgery and care of the bones, joints, tendons, and ligaments	Any broken bone, torn cartilage and ligaments, ruptured spinal discs
Neurosurgeons	Surgery of the brain and nervous system	Brain aneurysms, ruptured spinal discs
Otolaryngologist (Ear, Nose and Throat – ENT surgery)	Surgery of the ear, nose and throat	Sinus surgery, rhinoplasty (nose jobs), tonsillectomy
Cardiac Surgeon or Cardio-Thoracic Surgeons	Heart surgery and surgery on the other organs and structures in the chest	Coronary artery bypass surgery (surgery to prevent heart attacks done to the blood vessels that supply the heart with blood)
Vascular Surgeon	Blood vessel surgery except for those within the brain and heart (typically performed by a neurosurgeon or cardiothoracic surgeon)	Varicose vain removal, aortic aneurysm surgery
Bariatric Surgeon	Weight reduction surgery	Lap bands, gastric bypass surgery
Urologist	Urinary system – kidney, bladder of both sexes, and reproductive system of men – prostate, testicles, penis	Kidney stone removal, male impotence, prostate cancer
Colorectal Surgeon	Surgery of the colon	Colon cancer

| Plastic Surgery | Surgery and procedures on surface structures – skin, soft tissues, facial structures | Rhinoplasty /nose jobs, liposuction, breast reconstruction after mastectomy |

Mix of Medicine and Surgery-Based

Specialty	What they do	Examples of common scenarios/conditions treated
Obstetrics and Gynecology	Women's health and primary care for women of reproductive age	Prenatal care, uterine fibroids, ovarian cysts, cervical cancer
Emergency Medicine	Stabilize individuals with serious illness	Any sudden life- or limb-threatening illness or trauma
Dermatology	Diseases of the skin	Eczema, psoriasis, skin cancers
Ophthalmologists	Eye diseases and surgery of the eye and eyelids	Glaucoma, cataracts, retinal detachment

Other

Specialty	What they do	Examples of common scenarios/conditions treated
Radiology	Interpret imaging studies	Interpret X-rays, CT scans, ultrasounds, MRIs
Interventional Radiology	Subset of radiologists who perform image-guided procedures	Stent placement, uterine fibroid treatment

Pathology	Microscopic analysis of body tissues to help in disease diagnoses	Oversee laboratory tests like blood counts; help in the diagnosis of various cancers and blood diseases
Physical Medicine and Rehabilitation	Care for people in the recovery phase of major illnesses	Rehabilitation after a stroke or major illness, surgery or trauma; may care for people with chronic pain
Psychiatrists	Care for mental health-related conditions	Bipolar disease, depression, anxiety, schizophrenia
Anesthesiologist/Pain Specialists	Pain control specialists	Administer anesthesia prior to surgical procedures to produce pain relief and unawareness; pain specialists care for people with chronic pain
Palliative Care Specialists	Prevent and lessen suffering during an illness	Prescribe treatments to control pain and uncomfortable symptoms, assist with difficult medical decisions – focus is on quality of life

This is not an exhaustive list, and there is occasionally overlap between the various specialists (figure 5-2). Internists and family medicine doctors sometimes overlap since they both provide primary care to adults. Allergists and pulmonologists both treat asthma. Anesthesiologists, palliative medicine specialists, and physical medicine and rehabilitation doctors all treat chronic pain. In the world of surgery, many surgeons also overlap on the parts of the body on which they operate – neurosurgeons and orthopedic surgeons both treat the spine; vascular surgeons and thoracic surgeons both operate on blood vessels in the chest; plastic surgeons operate on the ears and nose along with ENT doctors, the eyelids and brows along with ophthalmologists, and the skin along with dermatologists; both OB-GYNs and urologists operate on a women's bladder; and general surgeons and colorectal surgeons both operate on the colon. Finally, interventional radiologists are specialists within radiology who use image-guided procedures with catheter wires and cameras to diagnose and treat diseases in nearly every organ system. They have developed techniques that often remove the need for traditional surgery. For example, instead of surgically removing fibroids in women, growths on the uterus, interventional radiologists can use a catheter wire to destroy the blood supply to the fibroid, thus making it shrivel and die.

Figure 5-2 Doctors Who Overlap in the Services They Provide

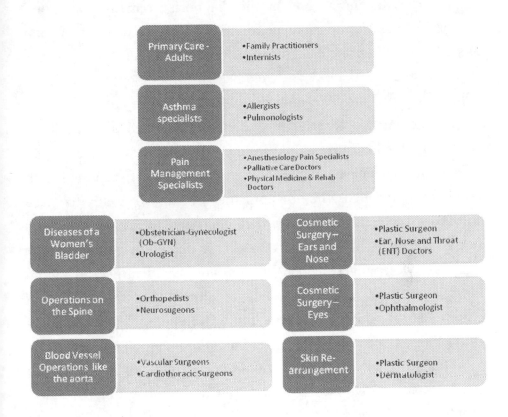

With all these allopathic doctors to choose from, it may be overwhelming when faced with choosing the right one for you. Later in the chapter, we will review the ways to choose an individual allopathic doctor and make sure that choice is right for you.

What Illnesses and Conditions Respond Well to Allopathy?

Because allopathy is the most common type of medicine practiced, many people have had experience with allopathic doctors, and some of it has not always been positive. Some concerns with allopathic medicine relate more to the attitudes and behaviors of certain doctors and not to the discipline of allopathy. At its best, allopathic medicine is good at the diagnosis of many conditions, especially ones that need to be identified and acted upon as soon as possible. It employs a high degree of scientific scrutiny to ensure that the treatments used are effective for what they are intended. Allopathy can provide immediate relief from acute and also life-threatening problems, usually using well researched medically or surgically based treatments. Treatments are often immediate in their effects and convenient to take. These treatments can keep the health condition controlled while or until the consumer is ready to make the necessary lifestyle changes that may lead to improved health. For individuals who are not yet ready or unable to commit to the daily lifestyle changes needed to improve their health or for whom lifestyle approaches are not effective, allopathic medicine offers a wide range of options to control the unpleasant effects of a variety of conditions.

There are, of course, limitations to allopathic medicine, which is why many individuals now seek out and choose other kinds of practitioners. Here are some of the limitations: Allopathy does not excel at curing problems once they have gotten into the chronic stage – beyond the first three months. In addition, for diseases of the brain and nervous system – dementia, Lou Gehrig's disease/ ALS, Parkinson's – there are currently few effective treatments. Treatments for cancers, especially once they have spread to other places in the body, often have severe side effects, are difficult to endure. Many treatments for illnesses of any type only slow how fast the disease progresses. Medications in particular have their own problems. Side effects of many prescribed medications, especially when taking several together, can range from irritating to life-threatening. Finally, challenges exist with the way the system of allopathic medicine is practiced. There is often poor communication within the system. When poor communication exists between doctors and doctors and other health-care professionals, errors can often occur. When there is poor communication between doctors and consumers, not only can serious errors occur, but also consumers often feel dissatisfied with their treatment. Health-care reform legislation is fueling efforts to reorganize allopathic medicine to address some of these shortcomings. We will cover some of these changes in the next chapter and how they affect you, the consumer.

Osteopathic Medicine

What They Do: Osteopathic medicine practitioners are also known as doctors of osteopathy (DO). They provide care that is just like that provided in allopathic medicine – prescription drugs and surgery for treatment and the use of technology to diagnose disease and evaluate injury. They treat the same illnesses and provide primary and specialty care, just like MDs. The main difference is the use of manipulation to restore the body's natural alignment. The founder of osteopathy, Dr. Andrew Taylor Still, who lived in the 1800s, wanted to promote the body's innate ability to heal itself through a system of diagnosis and therapy known as osteopathic manipulative medicine (OMM). OMM is based on the belief that most diseases are related to problems in the body' system of muscles, nerves, and bones and that restoring the proper relationship of these structures to each other will restore their proper function. With structure restored, the body's own natural healing powers will be able to restore full health.

Figure 5-3 *Osteopathic Manipulative Medicine (OMM)*
Techniques

OMM introduced a series of techniques that you may
come across if you visit a DO or other practitioner that
uses physical manipulation. Some of these techniques are:

- craniosacral therapy – the manipulating of the
  bones of the skull to restore balance to the whole
  body
- myofascial release – massage of muscle and
  other tissues designed to improve blood flow and
  drainage and thus loosen and relax tight painful
  tissues
- muscle energy technique – tensing a muscle in
  order to stretch it and the accompanying joint
  fully; used to treat stiff and painful joints and
  muscles
- counterstrain – passive stretch of a muscle to
  relieve pain
- visceral manipulation; gentle massage of the
  internal organs by the practitioner to relax them
  and reestablish proper alignment

Although the training of osteopathic physicians in the United
States is very similar to that of their MD counterparts, it also includes
training in OMM. A good question to ask if you are considering an
osteopath is if they use OMM in their clinical practice. Access the
website of the American Osteopathic Association to locate a licensed
DO in your area who has been trained in an approved medical school
or teaching hospital. Just as with allopathic doctors, most insurance
companies, Medicaid and Medicare cover visits.

What Illnesses and Conditions Respond Well to Osteopathy?

The best scientific evidence shows that osteopathic manipulation is most effective for back and neck pain. In fact, you may be able to reduce the amount of pain medication you are taking for back pain if you receive osteopathic manipulation as part of your therapy. Preliminary evidence also shows that it may be helpful for:

- Ankle injuries
- Asthma
- Fibromyalgia
- Tennis elbow
- Chronic obstructive pulmonary disease (COPD)
- Recovery after surgery
- Menstrual pain
- Depression
- Irritable bowel syndrome (IBS)

Manipulation can cause temporary increases in pain, headache, or fatigue. Rarely, stroke and spinal injury have been reported following manipulation of the neck. If you have a disease of the bones – like a broken bone, bone cancer, bone infection, damaged ligaments, rheumatoid arthritis of the neck, or osteoporosis – you should avoid osteopathic manipulation. Osteopathic manipulation is also not recommended for people who recently underwent joint surgery or for people taking an anticoagulant (blood thinning) medication, such as aspirin or warfarin (Coumadin).

Naturopathic Medicine

What They Do: Naturopathic medicine is based on the belief that the human body has an innate healing ability. Naturopathic medicine seeks to find the least invasive measures necessary for symptom improvement or resolution and thus minimize use of surgery and prescription medications. Naturopathic doctors (NDs) focus on diet, exercise, lifestyle changes, and natural therapies to enhance the body's ability to ward off and combat disease. Naturopathic physicians follow three main principles:

- Use low-risk procedures and healing compounds – such as dietary supplements and herbal extracts – with few or no side effects.
- When possible, do not suppress symptoms, which are the body's efforts to self-heal. For example, fever, as a response to bacterial infection, is the body's way of destroying the bacteria, so a naturopath would not try to suppress it unless the body temperature was dangerously high.
- Customize each diagnosis and treatment plan to fit each individual.

Although the phrase was coined in the late 1800s, a renewed interest in naturopathic medicine took place in the 1970s. There are two kinds of practitioners – naturopathic doctors (ND) and traditional naturopaths. Naturopathic doctors consider themselves as primary-care providers, and in addition to various natural approaches, they prescribe drugs, perform minor surgery, and apply other conventional medical approaches to their practice. They also receive training in *acupuncture* and *traditional Chinese medicine*, *botanical medicine, homeopathy*, nature cure (a range of therapies based upon exposure to natural elements), *nutrition, physical medicine*, and *psychological counseling*. In the U.S., currently seventeen states (Alaska, Arkansas, California, Colorado, Connecticut, Hawaii, Idaho, Kansas, Maine, Minnesota, Montana, New Hampshire, North Dakota, Oregon, Utah, Vermont, Washington), the District of Columbia, Puerto Rico, and the U.S. Virgin Islands have licensing laws for naturopathic doctors. In these states, getting licensed requires graduation from one of the six four-year accredited naturopathic medical schools and passing a board examination (NPLEX) after graduation.

Traditional naturopaths have to follow the three main principles listed above but totally avoid the use of drugs, surgery, disease-specific treatments, or the practice of conventional medicine. The level of naturopathic training varies among traditional naturopaths in the United States. Traditional naturopaths may complete non-degree certificate programs or undergraduate degree programs. In states that license naturopathic doctors, traditional naturopaths cannot call themselves NDs and often use the term "naturopathic consultant." If you want to choose an ND, make sure they have graduated from a program approved by the American Association of Naturopathic Physicians (AANP). Treatment by naturopathic doctors is not covered by many insurance policies, including those offered through Medicare and Tricare. States that license naturopathic doctors as primary-care providers may provide coverage on Medicaid programs and may require that care provided by a licensed ND be covered by insurance. The best thing to do is to check with your insurance company in their policy.

Some of the more common treatments used by NDs include:

- Nutritional counseling
- Herbal medicine – including botanical medicines, vitamins, minerals, and allergy treatments
- Homeopathic medicine – giving very small doses of highly diluted substances believed to cause symptoms similar the condition being treated
- Acupuncture – using small needles to stimulate the flow of blocked energy in the body, thereby treating illness and pain.
- Hydrotherapy (water therapy) – these therapies include drinking natural spring water, alternating hot and cold applications, and water exercise, all of which are thought to stimulate healing and strengthen the immune system.
- Physical medicine – the use of touch, hot and cold compresses, electric currents, and sound waves to manipulate the muscles, bones, and spine.
- Detoxification – this therapy removes toxins from the body by fasting, using enemas, and drinking lots of water.
- Spirituality – personal spiritual development is encouraged as part of an overall health program.
- Lifestyle and psychological counseling – an ND may use hypnosis, guided imagery, or other counseling methods as part of a treatment plan.

What Illnesses and Conditions Respond Well to Naturopathy?

The effectiveness of naturopathy as a whole system has not been systematically evaluated. One 2008 study did show that in a group of seventy warehouse workers treated for back pain with a *naturopathic approach* – incorporating acupuncture, exercise and dietary advice, relaxation training, and a back-care booklet – was more cost effective than the employer's usual patient education program in treating low-back pain. Naturopaths treat both acute and chronic conditions, and they will work in conjunction with the treatment plans of allopathic or osteopathic doctors. If you choose to go this route, it is critical to tell all your providers what treatments you are receiving and foster communication among all of them.

Integrative Medical Physicians

What They Do: Integrative medicine is the practice of marrying allopathic or osteopathic medicine with the approach and practices that many naturopathic or other complementary medical traditions use. Integrative physicians will often combine therapies and treatment approaches from different traditions. Although a relatively recent field, states such as Texas have begun to establish practice guidelines for MDs or DOs who integrate alternative and complementary medicine into their practice. There is great variety in both the type of training in alternative practices that physicians get as well as the kinds of practices they choose to employ in their practice. Each integrative physician is unique. However, once trained, they continue to be known as MDs or DOs but often use terms such as "holistic," "natural," or "integrative" to describe their practice. The American Naturopathic Medical Association (ANMA) and American Naturopathic Medical Certification and Accreditation Board (ANMCAB) has recognition and certification programs for medical doctors (MD) and doctors of osteopathic medicine (DO) who have supplemented their education with naturopathic studies and integrate naturopathy into their practice.

What Illnesses and Conditions Respond Well to Integrative Medicine?

Because integrative medicine is still an emerging field, there have not yet been well-done studies looking at how it measures up. Practices still vary widely. However, if you are interested in finding a physician who combines a conventional allopathic approach with various elements of complementary medicine, you can seek out an integrative practitioner. Start out with understanding what complementary practices that doctor uses, their training and experience in these practices, and any evidence they can provide of how well they work. Many integrative practitioners make efforts to involve you in your care and taking a proactive approach to health. In addition, they commonly structure their practices so that visits can last more than the standard ten to fifteen minutes at conventional doctor's office, especially for the first visit.

Finding One in Your Area: The American Academy for Advancement in Medicine (ACAM) and the American Association of Integrative Medicine are both professional societies for integrative physicians. Their websites feature a physician locator you can use to find an integrative physician near you.

Chiropractic Medicine

What They Do: Chiropractic medicine, started in 1895, is concerned with the diagnosis, treatment and prevention of disorders of the *neuro-musculoskeletal* system – nerves, muscles, and bones – and the effects of these disorders on general health. Chiropractic's goal is to ensure the spine is in alignment in order to relieve stress on the nervous system. Chiropractic's thinking is that by relieving stress on the spinal nerves, which travel to all parts of the body, the entire body will function better. The main chiropractic treatment technique involves manual therapy, including manipulation of the spine, other joints, and soft tissues. Treatment also includes exercises and health and lifestyle counseling. Manual treatment takes place on a specially designed table where the chiropractor moves a joint to the end of its range, then applies a low force thrust. Other treatment techniques include massage and heat and ice therapies. Although chiropractors now use more gentle manipulations, the vast majority of chiropractic adjustments still use some variation of the thrust technique. Chiropractic uses some of the same techniques as other manual-therapy professions, including massage therapy, osteopathy, and physical therapy.

Chiropractic is widely accepted – all fifty states, the District of Columbia, Puerto Rico, and the U.S. Virgin Islands recognize it as a health-care profession and have state or territory licensing requirements in order to practice. The number of classroom hours required for a doctor of chiropractic (DC) degree is similar to that for a medical degree. To find the licensed chiropractors in your area you can access the website of the largest association of chiropractors, the American Chiropractic Association. Most employer-based health care plans cover at least part of the cost of chiropractic and Medicare, Medicaid, and worker's compensation fully reimburse for chiropractic care.

What Conditions Are Treated Effectively with Chiropractic?

Low-back pain is the most common reason people seek out the care of chiropractors. Chiropractic has been shown to be effective for acute and chronic low-back pain, neck pain, and headaches. Preliminary evidence suggests it may also help frozen shoulder, tennis elbow and other sports injuries, carpal tunnel syndrome, otitis media (ear infection), digestive problems, menstrual and premenstrual pain, attention deficit hyperactivity disorder (ADHD), and asthma. The same precautions that exist for osteopathic manipulation also apply to chiropractic manipulation. Minor but common side effects of spinal manipulative therapy (SMT) may include local or radiating discomfort, headache, or tiredness. There are risks associated with joint manipulation, especially spinal joints. Rare but potentially serious side effects, include strokes, spinal disc herniation, vertebral and rib fractures, and cauda equina syndrome, a type of spinal nerve damage.

Homoepathic Medicine

What They Do: Homeopathy seeks to stimulate the body's ability to heal itself by giving very small doses of highly diluted substances believed to cause symptoms similar to the condition being treated. The therapy was developed by German physician Samuel Hahnemann at the end of the eighteenth century. Homeopathy works off two fundamental beliefs. The first is that "like cures like" – substances that cause a set of symptoms can be used to cure diseases that produce similar symptoms. The other belief is the "law of minimum dose," which states that the lower the dose of the medication, the greater its effectiveness. Dilution often continues until none of the original substance remains, and no pharmacologic effect is present. Modern homeopathic practitioners believe that *water has a memory*, allowing homeopathic preparations to work without any of the original diluted substance.

Homeopaths examine aspects of the individual's symptoms, physical and psychological state, and consult homeopathic reference books known as "repertories" to select a remedy. Homeopaths recommend against practices such as vaccinations, antimalarial drugs, and antibiotics. However, these recommendations have been criticized by conventional medicine as not being based on researched information.

Practitioners of homeopathy have varied backgrounds and credentials. Currently, there are no uniform licensing or professional standards for the practice of homeopathy in the United States. The licensing of homeopaths varies from state to state. Currently, licensure as a homeopathic physician is available only to medical doctors (MD) and doctors of osteopathy (DO) in Arizona, Connecticut, and Nevada. Certification is available through the American Board of Homeo-therapeutics to medical doctors and doctors of osteopathic medicine (DOs) who have specialized in homeopathy (DHt indicates a doctor of homeopathy). Naturopathic doctors study homeopathy extensively as part of their medical training and some are certified by the Homeopathic Academy of Naturopathic Physicians (DHANP). In states that grant licenses to NDs, licensure includes homeopathy in their scope of practice. Finally, California, Rhode Island, and Minnesota give unlicensed health-care practitioners the freedom to engage in "complementary and alternative health-care practices," and this could involve homeopathy. Any practitioner of homeopathy can apply for Certification in Classical Homeopathy (CCH).

Depending on state law, unlicensed practitioners are required to disclose their training and qualifications to their clients and not represent themselves as a doctor. Insurance companies are more likely to cover homeopathy when the person providing the service is a licensed health-care professional, such as an MD, ND or DO who also practices homeopathy.

To find a homeopathic provider in your area, you can contact one of several organizations, including the Council for Homeopathic Certification, the National Center for Homeopathy, the American Association of Naturopathic Physicians, the North American Society of Homeopaths, or the Homeopathic Educational Services.

What Illnesses and Conditions Respond Well to Homeopathy?

There are not many published analyses supporting the use of homeopathy as an effective treatment for any specific condition. A few studies have reported positive results from homeopathic treatments, but to date, these results have not been replicated or seen in higher quality trials. Due to the limited amount of research, more high-quality research studies are needed on both the safety and the effectiveness of these remedies. Homeopathy is difficult to study using current scientific methods for a number of reasons. Highly diluted substances (known as ultrahigh dilutions or UHDs) cannot be readily measured, making it difficult to design or replicate studies. In addition, very little standardization exists in homeopathic treatments. Literally hundreds of different homeopathic remedies exist, which can be prescribed in a variety of different dilutions, and are used to treat thousands of symptoms.

People use homeopathy for a range of health concerns, including prevention of illness. Common uses include the treatment of allergies, asthma, chronic fatigue syndrome, depression, digestive disorders, ear infections, colds, headaches, and skin rashes. Homeopathic remedies are regulated in the same manner as nonprescription drugs, but because they have little or no active ingredients, they do not have to undergo the same safety and efficacy testing. The U.S. Food and Drug Administration (FDA) does require that homeopathic remedies meet certain legal standards for strength, purity, and packaging. The labels on the remedies must include at least one medical problem to be treated, a list of ingredients, the dilution, and safety instructions. In addition, if a homeopathic remedy claims to treat a serious disease such as cancer, it needs to be sold by prescription. Only products for minor health problems that usually go away on their own, like a cold or insomnia, can be sold without a prescription. Health food stores and some pharmacies sell homeopathic remedies for a variety of problems. Remedies are usually taken for no more than two to three days. In some cases, daily dosing may be prescribed.

Homeopathy should not be used to postpone seeing a doctor about a medical problem, or treat conditions that require immediate relief of symptoms. You should never treat a life-threatening illness with homeopathy alone. Evaluate if the homeopathic remedy you are considering has been studied for the health condition you need treated. In addition, it is advisable to understand the training and experience of the practitioner you are considering. Women who are pregnant or nursing or people who are thinking of using homeopathy to treat a child, should first consult their health-care provider.

Acupuncture and Traditional Chinese Medicine (TCM)

What They Do: Acupuncture has been practiced for thousands of years in Asian countries and is one of the key components of traditional Chinese medicine (TCM). TCM thinks of the body as a large electrical grid, with energy or qi (pronounced *chee*) circulating throughout it all the time. This qi runs through channels called meridians, similar to electricity going through electrical wires. The meridians connect energy centers located at various points throughout the body. At birth, these energy centers are all filled with qi. We all start out life with a set amount of qi inherited from our parents, which we use up in the process of living. When it is all gone, death occurs. However, qi is replenished daily through the fuels we take in such as food, air, and water. Depending on the quality of fuels we take in, our qi can be enhanced and less of the limited original qi is needed to sustain life. Disease results when the flow of qi or energy throughout the body is blocked due to an internal imbalance. Conversely, health occurs when blockages are eliminated, and qi is flowing easily. There are over two thousand points along the meridians where the energy is close to the skin surface and can be easily accessed. Acupuncturists unblock qi by penetrating the skin at these acupuncture points with thin, solid, metallic needles known as acupuncture needles.

The National Certification Commission for Acupuncture and Oriental Medicine certifies acupuncturists (Dipl Ac) and practitioners of Chinese herbal medicine (Dipl CH) who pass a qualifying exam. Other medical practitioners may perform acupuncture as well, most often naturopathic physicians and oriental medical doctors (OMDs). Increasingly, medical doctors and nurse practitioners are integrating it into their practice. Most states require acupuncturists to be licensed and confer a title (LAc). The American Academy of Medical Acupuncture can provide a list of licensed physicians in your area who are also trained to perform acupuncture.

What Illnesses and Conditions Respond Well to Acupuncture?

Acupuncture is particularly effective for relief of pain and lessening of nausea and vomiting after surgery or chemotherapy. In addition, both the World Health Organization and the National Institutes of Health recognize that acupuncture can be a helpful part of a treatment plan for many illnesses including addiction (such as alcoholism), asthma, bronchitis, carpal tunnel syndrome, constipation, diarrhea, facial tics, fibromyalgia, headaches, irregular menstrual cycles, polycystic ovarian syndrome, low-back pain, menopausal symptoms, menstrual cramps, osteoarthritis, sinusitis, irritable bowel syndrome, stroke rehabilitation, tendonitis, tennis elbow, and urinary problems such as incontinence. You can safely combine acupuncture with prescription drugs and other conventional treatments, but it is important for your prescribing doctor to be aware of and monitor how your acupuncture treatment may be interacting with conventional therapies. The number of acupuncture treatment sessions needed varies with the condition you are getting treated. For example, pain from a recent ankle sprain may require fewer treatments than longstanding migraine headaches.

Figure 5-4: Common diagnoses for which insurance companies will cover acupuncture

Chronic low-back pain

Migraine headache

Pain from osteoarthritis of the knee or hip (when done with other conventional treatments)

Nausea and vomiting related to pregnancy, surgery, or chemotherapy

Dental pain after a procedure

Temporomandibular joint disease (TMJ) – a disorder of the jaw

Insurance companies are increasingly covering most of, if not all, the cost of acupuncture treatments. The best course of action is to check what your policy offers. A few policies may cover the cost of treatments no matter what the diagnosis is, but many limit coverage to few diagnoses.

Ayurveda

What They Do: Originating in India almost five thousand years ago, Ayurveda, or the "science of life," is considered one of the oldest systems of medicine in the world. The basic principle of Ayurveda is to prevent and treat illness by maintaining balance in the body, mind, and spirit through proper drinking, diet, and lifestyle and the use of herbal remedies. Ayurveda teaches that the entire universe, including our bodies, our food, and the environment is made up of the following five elements: earth, water, fire, air, and space. Each entity is composed of these elements in its own unique proportions. Our particular elemental makeup or constitution (*prakuti*) dictates what balance looks like for each of us. Many factors influence which constitution we are born with: heredity, our parents' health at our conception, the environment in our mother's womb, astrology, and related to reincarnation, what we brought from our past lives. Our constitution is with us from birth and *never* changes. There are three main energy types called doshas – *pitta* (bile), *kapha* (phlegm), and *vata* (wind). These doshas combine in unique ways in each of us to give each individual a characteristic energy pattern. Each *dosha* is a combination of two of the five elements earth, water, fire, air, and space. The combinations are as follows:

- *Pitta* = Fire + Water – Pitta energy controls the body's metabolic systems, including digestion, absorption, nutrition, and temperature. In balance, pitta leads to contentment and intelligence. Out of balance, pitta can cause ulcers and arouse anger. Pitta predominant people have sharp facial features and intellect. They are usually of medium build, have strong appetites, and have good digestion. They tend to run hot and may easily perspire and become red in the face. Pittas have focused concentration but can be easily frustrated and angered. They love spicy food and acidic foods that are primarily fire and water.

- *Kapha* = Water + Earth – Kapha energy controls growth in the body. It supplies water to all body parts, moisturizes the skin, and maintains the immune system. In balance, kapha is expressed as love and forgiveness. Out of balance, kapha leads to insecurity and envy. Kapha types are usually larger and heavier, and their skin appears milky and smooth. Their features are round and wide, and their hair tends to be voluminous. They are grounded people with strength and endurance. Kaphas can be nurturing and loving but may also become greedy and possessive of things and people. They tend to be lethargic and may have a slow metabolism. This type of person prefers dairy products and rich foods that are primarily earth and water.

- *Vata* = Air + Space – Energy that controls bodily functions associated with motion, including blood circulation, breathing, blinking, and heartbeat. When vata energy is balanced, there is creativity and vitality. Out of balance, vata produces fear and anxiety. Vata predominant people tend to be lean, with dry skin and coarse hair and tend to have irregular bodily functions, like irregular appetite and elimination. They tend to be creative, are very busy, prefer to do several things at once, have nervous habits, and can be easily distracted. They prefer raw food because it is mostly air and space.

Figure 5-5: Examples of Ayurvedic Treatments

A vata aggravation with symptoms of gas, bloating, constipation, and irregular appetite, would be worse with eating vata foods like salads and beans. A treatment would be to eat foods possessing the opposite qualities: warm, heavy, oily foods like stews and soups with warming spices.

Excess pitta can show up as hyperacidity, skin rashes, or inflammatory conditions, so avoiding hot, spicy, oily foods may be prescribed. Foods that are cooling, sweet and bitter, like cucumbers, watermelon, most legumes, and most dairy products would be the treatment.

For excess kapha-like symptoms of sinus congestion or water retention, you might be told to avoid dairy and fats and choose raw or steamed leafy vegetables and grains such as buckwheat and millet.

An individual may be any one or a combination of these types. Many things can disturb the energy balance, such as stress, an unhealthy diet, the weather, and strained family relationships. The disturbance shows up as disease. Ayurvedic practitioners assess your dosha, any imbalances present, and prescribe treatments to bring the doshas back into balance. Ayurveda teaches that "like increases like." In terms of diet, this means that foods of vata nature will increase vata in the body and likewise for pitta and kapha.

Examples of treatments include prescribing foods that intensify or oppose a particular dosha; Yoga, mantras, and breathing exercises for stress reduction; herbal oils for the skin to increase blood circulation and draw toxins out of the body through the skin; detoxification through methods that cause sweat, bowel movements, and even vomit; and herbal medicines to restore dosha balance.

To find qualified Ayurvedic practitioners in your area, contact the National Institute of Ayurvedic Medicine (NIAM). Although none of the fifty states offer a license to practice Ayurveda, there are several institutions across the United States that have educational programs that issue a certificate of clinical Ayurveda.

What Illnesses and Conditions Respond Well to Ayurveda?

Most ayurveda treatments for specific conditions have not yet been tested in rigorous scientific studies or have not been shown to be beneficial. For example, a systematic review of Ayurveda treatments for rheumatoid arthritis concluded that there was insufficient evidence, as most of the trials were not done properly, and the one high-quality trial showed no benefits. A review of Ayurveda and heart disease concluded that the evidence for Ayurveda was not convincing, though some herbs seemed promising in reversing the thickening of artery walls known as atherosclerosis.

On the other hand, certain specific treatments within Ayurveda have shown promise. Yoga, for example, has been shown to improve circulation and digestion and to reduce blood pressure, cholesterol levels, anxiety, and chronic pain. Certain individual herbal remedies suggest promise, but high-quality studies are still lacking. Some examples include guggul *(Commiphora mukul)* and Fenugreek seeds *(Trigonella foenum graecum)* for cholesterol lowering; Common sage *(Salvia officinalis)* for memory in indviduals with Alzheimer's disease; and the antioxidant effects of Neem, a herb used for detoxification to remove excess pitta and kapha. Because Ayurvedic herbs may interact with medications prescribed by a medical doctor, it is essential that your doctor know you if are considering Ayurvedic herbs. In addition, there have been concerns, highlighted by several studies, about the practice of adding toxic heavy metals such as lead, mercury, and arsenic to herbal treatments. Although the government of India ruled that Ayurvedic products must specify their metallic content on the label, there is not clear evidence yet of effective quality control of Ayurvedic medicines. Ask your health-care provider about choosing quality supplements for you and your family.

Be Familiar with Alternative Treatments

So we have gone through general types of medical systems you may encounter which offer primary assessment and care of health concerns. In addition to this broad overview of practitioners, I also wanted to provide you with a description of some additional therapies they may employ or recommend. These therapies are becoming more popular in various medical practices, hospitals, and in the treatment of chronic conditions. Some have been more extensively studied than others, but when used, they can be included as part of a integrated approach to treatment by a variety of medical practitioners working together.

Cognitive Behavioral Therapy

Cognitive behavioral therapy (CBT) is a type of mental health therapy based on the idea that our thoughts cause our feelings and behaviors, not external things, like people, situations, and events. In this way, we can overcome persistent challenges by changing our thinking, behavior, and emotional responses even if the situation does not change. CBT generally requires fewer sessions than other types of therapy to get results and is done in a structured way that deals directly with specific challenges. A mental health counselor helps you to become aware of inaccurate or negative thinking. You can thereby view challenging situations more clearly and respond to them in a more effective way.

To find a therapist, you can get a referral from a doctor, health insurance plan, employee assistance program (EAP), or a trusted source. The American Psychological Association website also offers a psychologist locator service. A therapist should be a licensed counselor, psychologist, or other mental health provider experienced in cognitive behavioral therapy. Some health plans do cover mental health counseling and CBT in particular, so if you have health insurance, check for coverage and how many sessions are specified. Therapists may also have various payment options available.

What Can It Be Used For?

Given what we know about the role that our response to stress plays in the appearance of illness, CBT is one tool that can help us manage or response to stress and potentially improve our physical health. When combined with other therapies, it can be a useful tool to address depression, anxiety, low self-esteem, addictions, phobias, anger, grief, emotional trauma, and relationship conflict. CBT can also be used to manage chronic physical symptoms, such as pain, sleeplessness, or fatigue.

Prior to your first session, it would be good to spend some time prioritizing the issues you want to address. To get the most out of your sessions, it is best to spend time between sessions on the home exercises that the CBT therapist assigns.

Reiki

Reiki is a healing practice that originated in Japan that means "universal life energy." Reiki practitioners place their hands lightly on or just above the person receiving treatment with the goal of facilitating the person's own healing response. Reiki is used to promote overall well-being and to get relief from disease-related symptoms and the side effects of conventional medical treatments. Reiki has been used by people with anxiety, chronic pain, HIV/AIDS, and other health conditions as well as by people recovering from surgery or experiencing side effects from cancer treatments. Reiki has also been given to people who are dying (and to their families and caregivers) to help impart a sense of peace. The practice of Reiki requires training, but currently, training and certification for Reiki practitioners are not formally regulated.

What Can Reiki Be Used For?

Research is under way to learn more about how Reiki may work, its possible effects on health, and diseases and conditions for which it may be helpful. Studies that have looked at the effect on wound healing, stress, chronic illness, blood counts, anxiety, and pain either were not well designed or found no influence of Reiki in these conditions. However, energy medicine researchers assert that Reiki is difficult to study in clinical trials. This is because in clinical trials, there is always a comparison group who gets a different treatment than the one being tested, in this case, Reiki. The comparison groups in Reiki trials always receive some form of "laying on of hands," usually from someone who is untrained in Reiki. However, energy medicines researchers assert that even inexperienced people will have some effect through energy fields, making it not a true baseline comparison. So until well-designed trials can be conducted, there is still no clear evidence on where Reiki is most effective.

Massage

Massage has been practiced as a healing therapy for centuries in nearly every culture around the world. In massage therapy, a therapist works with the muscles and other soft tissues of the body to improve health and well-being. There are nearly one hundred different massage and body work techniques. They vary based upon the amount of pressure used, area of body targeted, and goals of the therapy. Below are descriptions of the types of massage you are most likely to encounter in health care:

- **Craniosacral massage:** Gentle pressure is applied to the head and spine to correct imbalances and restore the flow of cerebrospinal fluid – the fluid that coats the brain and spinal cord.

- **Lymphatic massage:** Light, rhythmic strokes are used to improve the flow of lymph (body fluid that helps fight infection and disease) everywhere in the body. One type, manual lymphatic drainage (MLD), focuses on draining excess lymph from areas it has accumulated. It is commonly used on the legs and arms when circulation problems exist or lymph nodes have been surgically removed, such as in breast cancer.

- **Myofascial release:** Gentle pressure and body positioning are used to relax and stretch the muscles, fascia (connective tissue), and related structures. Trained physical therapists and massage therapists use this technique.

- **Reflexology:** The massaging of certain areas of the hands and feet that are believed to have direct connections to specific organs and structures throughout the body. The goal is relaxation and promotion of overall health.

- **Rolfing:** Pressure is applied to the fascia (the tissue covering and connecting muscles) to release tension and increase flexibility. The goal of this technique is to realign the body so that it functions better.

- **Shiatsu:** Shiatsu uses finger-and-hand pressure to target the same points acupuncturists treat with needles. The goals are to relieve pain and enhance health by improving the flow of qi energy through the body.

- **Swedish massage:** A variety of strokes and pressure techniques are used to enhance the flow of blood to the heart, remove waste products from the tissues, stretch ligaments and tendons, and ease physical and emotional tension.
- **Trigger-point massage:** Pressure is applied to trigger points (tender areas where the muscles have been damaged) to alleviate muscle spasms and pain.

Massage is usually offered by private practitioners in the community, but is slowly being integrated into a variety of health-care settings, such as skilled nursing facilities, hospice care facilities and hospitals. Certified massage therapists complete a training program of five hundred or more hours, take national board exams, and are licensed or registered in many states. To find a massage therapist in your area, visit the American Massage Therapy Association (AMTA) website.

What Can Massage Be Used For?

Massage is used for many musculoskeletal problems, such as low-back pain, and has been shown to be effective for it. Hand massage has been shown to help in persons with dementia with short-term reduction of agitated behavior and improvement of nutritional intake. More well-designed research is needed to determine how effective massage therapy is, which health problems improve the most from this technique, and whether it is more cost effective than other types of treatment.

Hypnosis

Recognized since 1958 by both the American Medical Association and the American Psychological Association as an effective medical procedure, hypnotherapy, as we know it today, was first practiced in the 1700s by an Austrian physician named Franz Anton Mesmer, the origin of the term *mesmerize.*

Hypnotherapists use special techniques that allow you as the participant to enter a trance state, similar to daydreaming. The person is fully conscious but tuning out other stimuli. You are relaxed, open to suggestion and intently focused, but only do what you agree to do. This is not the popular image of hypnosis where the hypnotherapist controls a person's decision-making.

Hypnosis is thought to work because it directly accesses to your subconscious or "behind the scenes" mind. Your subconscious mind is a huge storehouse of information that allows you to solve problems, automatically take care of actions like driving, and come up with new ideas. When you are awake, your conscious mind filters a lot of what happens on the subconscious level. But during hypnotherapy, the deep relaxation and focusing exercises allow the conscious mind takes a backseat to the subconscious mind. The subconscious is also the storehouse for memories, learned behaviors and the emotions that go with them. While you are open to suggestion and accessing the subconscious, the therapist can guide you to remember an event that led to a learned behavior, separate the emotion from the learned behavior, and replace unhealthy behaviors with new, healthier ones. After returning to usual awareness, the therapist asks you to reflect on the experience, and between sessions, you may be given exercises to do to reinforce the new behaviors. Hypnosis can thus teach you how to master your own awareness and thereby affect your own mental responses, perceptions and emotional states.

What Can Hypnosis Be Used For?

Research shows hypnotherapy is effective in the treatment of anxiety, many stress-related medical conditions, and pain management, especially cancer pain, postsurgical pain, and migraine. There are mixed findings of effectiveness for the treatment of habits and addictions such as overeating, smoking, and alcohol abuse. It has shown promise but requires more research in the following areas: bed wetting, nausea and vomiting, eating disorders, fibromyalgia, recurrence of ulcers, cystic fibrosis, insomnia, high blood pressure, birth pains, smoking cessation, and weight loss. Hypnosis might not be appropriate for a person who has seizures, psychotic symptoms, such as hallucinations and delusions, or for someone who is using drugs or alcohol. It should be used for pain control only after a doctor has done an evaluation for any physical disorder that might require medical or surgical treatment.

Be Familiar with Other Potential Team Members

When addressing an ongoing health condition, most individuals need more detailed, hands-on care than what happens in the doctor's office. There are several other kinds of health-care professionals who will help to provide these services as part of the doctor's treatment plan. They may also specifically help to coordinate the various services – medical, financial, daily living, and otherwise – that you and your family may need if limited by illness. Below are descriptions of some of the professionals who you may work with in the course of your treatment.

Dieticians/Nutritionists

Dietitians provide food and nutrition information to help people improve their health. Qualified dietitians also have the clinical training to modify diets to treat or help to manage conditions such as diabetes, heart disease, obesity, cancer, food allergies and intolerances. They can also advise on foods to help increase energy. A dietitian asks detailed questions about your current diet, exercise habits, general health and lifestyle in order to tailor an individualized eating plan. If you have a specific medical problem and have been referred to a dietitian by your doctor, the dietitian will work in close consultation with your doctor and may review blood and other test results to devise a suitable diet. You may be given written materials to take home. Follow-up appointments allow the dietitian to keep track of your progress and make adjustments to your eating plan as needed. The goal is to educate you on how to eat in a way that will keep you healthy so that you can choose the best food on your own.

Both dieticians and nutritionists advise on how food and nutrition impact health. However, the title *nutritionist* is not subject to professional regulation, and nutritionists can be wholly self-taught. The title of *dietitian* can be used only by those who have met specified professional requirements. When choosing a dietitian, look for someone with the qualification of registered dietitians

(RDs). You can find an RD through the website of the Academy for Nutrition and Dietetics.

Rehabilitative Therapists

Physical Therapists/Physiotherapists (PTs) diagnose and treat individuals of all ages who have illnesses or injuries that limit their abilities to move and perform their daily activities. Physical therapy is provided by *physical therapists*, who are licensed health-care professionals with a master's or doctorate degree in their field. Physical therapy can help with recovery after prolonged or severe illness or surgery. You doctor may refer you to a PT to heal after sudden injuries such as a broken bone or neck strain, to recover from procedures like knee replacement or heart surgery, to lessen chronic pain from conditions such as tendonitis or arthritis, to help children gain abilities not present due to developmental delay, to regain abilities lost due to chronic disease like heart failure or multiple sclerosis, or just to regain strength after a long and debilitating illness.

Regardless of the condition being treated, physical therapy may be used alone or with other treatments. The therapist's treatment plan will first address any pain and swelling and then move on to increasing flexibility, strength, and endurance. This is accomplished through specific exercises which you will be taught and asked to do at home, both between visits and after your formal therapy has ended. Faithful performance of the home exercises is essential to maintaining any gains you make during formal sessions. Physical therapy uses techniques such as massage, manipulation, traction, heat, cold, water, ultrasound, and electrical stimulation and also involves education on prevention of injury. After the first visit or two, it is normal to have some mild soreness or swelling, but if this persists or is bothersome, you should let your physical therapist know immediately.

You can find a qualified physical therapist at the website of the American Physical Therapy Association. If being referred by your doctor, your doctor may have a specific therapist in mind. Some states actually require a referral from a doctor, but others allow you to self-refer. It is important to check with your insurance company to see if they pay for physical therapy for your condition and what your copay amount will be. Many insurance plans will cover up to a certain number of visits without review. After that, they will want to know from your therapist that you are making progress before reimbursing for additional visits. If you are not making progress despite following all the recommendations of the therapist, it is best to be reevaluated by your doctor.

Occupational Therapists

Occupational therapy (OT) is the profession that helps people live as independently as possible by focusing on the daily living and work skills that have been impaired by a health condition. Occupational therapists (OTs) will evaluate your daily living needs as well as your home and work environments and provide recommendations. These recommendations may include making changes in those environments, suggesting strategies for new ways of doing things, or providing exercises to help you to better function. Daily activities can include personal care activities like dressing and eating, home skills like cooking, personal management skills like balancing a checkbook and keeping a schedule, and motor skills like driving or getting in and out of a car. OTs also address the use of assistive devices, posture, joint motion, protecting joints, overall strength and flexibility, and the most efficient way to perform tasks to conserve energy. Some examples where occupational therapy is useful include:

- addressing physical or developmental disabilities in children;
- facilitating return to work after a work-related injury;
- returning home after serious health conditions such as a stroke, heart attack, brain injury, or amputation;
- maximizing abilities in the face of debilitating conditions such as heart failure or dementia;
- helping individuals with mental illness acquire the skills to care for themselves; and
- addressing mental health issues associated with conditions such as post-traumatic stress or eating disorders.

Certification for occupational therapists is performed by the National Board for Certification in Occupational Therapy, and once certified, they are designated as Occupational Therapist Registered (OTR®). The American Occupational Therapy Association (AOTA) can help you find a qualified occupational therapist in your area who may specialize in your condition. Just as with physical therapy, it is advisable to check with your insurance company to see if they cover occupational therapy for your condition and what your copay amount will be. And also like physical therapy, health insurance companies may require a review of your progress before reimbursing for additional visits.

Speech Language Pathologists – Speech Therapists

Speech-Language Pathologists (SLPs), informally called speech therapists, specialize in communication disorders due to problems with speech, using and understanding language, voice, fluency, hearing, or reading and writing. Speech pathologists also work with difficulties related to swallowing food or drink. Speech pathologists would be involved in health issues such as feeding difficulties in an infant with a cleft palate, speech delay in child with hearing difficulties, loss of voice in teacher or singer due to overuse, severe brain injury, stuttering, poor swallowing due to stroke, and impaired communication due to disorders such as autism, cerebral palsy, and intellectual disability. Speech pathologists are licensed by the state in which they practice and are certified by the American Speech-Language-Hearing Association (ASHA), with a designation of CCC-SLP. Once again, check with your insurance company to see if they cover speech therapy for your condition, if they require a review of your progress before giving reimbursement for additional visits, and your copay amount.

Case Managers

A medical case manager links individuals with complex medical circumstances and their families with the appropriate resources to assure that their medical needs are met. The Case Management approach assumes that clients with complex and multiple needs are going to need services from a range of service providers. The goal is to make sure that everything is seamlessly coordinated. Case managers are often registered nurses, social workers, or occupational therapists who have earned additional certification in case management. A case manager listens to the client's story, develops a plan of care, provides choices, narrows down possibilities to come to a decision, does research, helps with paperwork, monitors changes in the client's situation, respects privacy, and maintains the client's routine and independence as much as possible.

The type of assistance a case manager provides largely depends on the setting. Health insurers or health plans often provide case management services to their clients who have complex medical needs. Examples of services that a case manager may provide through your health insurer include helping you to check your benefits, negotiating lower rates with providers who are not part of the plan's network, linking you to available community services, and coordinating referrals to specialists. By identifying members of the insurance plan who have major illnesses, contacting them, and actively coordinating their care, plans can reduce their expenses and improve the medical care their members receive. A typical scenario might be coordinating resources like occupational therapy and equipment like wheelchairs, ramps, and shower chairs for a member who had a stroke, now going home from the hospital. From the insurance company's perspective, if care is well coordinated, with an attention to good quality care, costs will be lower in the long run. For the member, it is a win-win situation because trying to bring all the moving pieces together can be time consuming and extremely difficult without prior experience.

Case managers also work for health-care providers/hospitals where they verify coverage and benefits with the health insurers to ensure the provider is appropriately paid, coordinate the services associated with discharge to a recovery facility or return home, provide health education, provide postcare follow-up, and coordinate services with other health-care providers. Case Managers often communicate with an individual and family, their physician(s), insurance company, community resources, care facilities, and providers of medical equipment to make sure the treatment plan is carried out seamlessly.

Case managers are also found at large companies with multiple employees. In this setting, they verify medical reasons for employee absences, follow up with employees after work absences due to poor health, provide health education, link employees with chronic illnesses with appropriate resources, provide on-site wellness programs, and assist employees to seek specialized treatment as needed.

Medical Social Workers

Medical social work (MSW) is a subdiscipline of *social work*, and their role often overlaps with hospital case managers. Medical social workers (MSWs) typically work in a hospital, skilled nursing facility or *hospice*, have a graduate degree in the field, and work with individuals and their families in need of social support. An MSW will assess how well an individual and their family are coping with their circumstances and intervene as necessary. Interventions may include connecting them to necessary resources and supports in the community, providing supportive counseling or grief counseling, or helping to expand and strengthen their network of social supports. The MSW plays a critical role helping individuals have proper postdischarge services as they leave the hospital. But of paramount importance, MSWs can act as advocates, especially in situations where they have identified problems that may compromise the discharge and put the individual at risk. For example, an MSW may identify that a frail elderly man who lives alone and is being discharged with home care services may not have the ability needed to direct a home care worker. It is then the MSW's job to recommend that the discharge plan be reassessed for the individual's safety and health needs and to suggest other options like a skilled nursing facility.

Takeaway Checklist

☐ Learning the purpose of each health-care professional is a key part of knowing what to expect from them when putting together your health-care team.

☐ A primary-care provider is good to have to provide continuity in the care you are getting – the more complex your condition, the more important this becomes.

☐ Various health-care practices – both alternative and conventional – excel at various skills. Knowing these can help you know who to tap when charting your particular path to wellness. Some therapies are needed to address the emotional components of an illness, address lifestyle, or to help prevent illness and maintain health. Others are better for physical recovery from illness, especially life-threatening ones.

☐ The key to interacting with more than one health-care professional is full disclosure – ensure each knows the other practitioners and treatments you are receiving.

☐ When you have a serious illness or complex condition, you may require a health-care team that involves members other than doctors such as medical social workers, case managers, nutritionists, and rehabilitation therapists. Knowing the roles of these other team members can help you get the most out of working with them.

Proactively Choose the Right Provider for You

The good physician treats the disease; the great physician treats the patient who has the disease.

– William Osler

In medical school, we were taught to examine patients by an experienced doctor in small groups of two to four students. A cardiologist taught me and my classmate Richard how to examine a patient's heart and blood vessels. Richard and I would travel over to his office once a week, and he would teach us what heart-related questions to ask, how to listen to the heart, and how to feel for pulses. He would then have us examine his office patients, most of whom were from inner-city Oakland, California. He never appeared to ask their permission. He would then insist that we report our findings to him in front of the patient while also commenting on how reliable we thought the information was that we got from them – again, in front of the patient. If our assessment of their reliability was too generous, he would fiercely correct us and say, "She's a terrible historian." One day, Richard examined an elderly lady who had circulatory problems that resulted in weak pulses in her feet. Richard, however, was able to detect some pulsations in her feet. He dutifully started off reporting his findings of the entire exam to the cardiologist. But when he got to the foot exam and reported feeling a pulse, he was immediately and rudely stopped. "What? This woman has no pulses in her feet! She hasn't had foot pulses in years," he bellowed. "Don't you ever say you feel something that isn't there! Now you examine her again, and I will be back in five minutes to hear your report!" And he stormed out of the room. Richard and I stood shell-shocked, intimidated at this display. When Richard started the task of reexamining her, the lady looked at him and said, "It's okay, baby. My foot doctor feels pulses. Don't worry, you'll be a good doctor . . . one day."

S TUDIES HAVE SHOWN that individuals with a regular source of care get better care even when they are uninsured. Additionally, it is also proven that it is hard to get a doctor's appointment at short notice when cold-calling a doctor you have never visited. Choosing a doctor, therefore, is an important step in being proactive about your health. You will trust this person for his or her expertise, advice, and treatment that will affect the quality of your life. However, all practitioners are not equally skilled, and not every physician will be a good fit. For example, the cardiologist above did not afford those whom he treated with due respect. Not only did he devalue what his patient had to say, but he had us, as medical students, talk to them without first getting their permission. He also did not treat them as partners in co-managing their health. The patient, whom we had the privilege of examining, was much more aware about her body than her doctor gave her credit for.

Unfortunately, there are many dissatisfied people who keep going back to doctors they do not like, thinking they have no choice. When an individual gets stuck with a doctor in whom he or she lacks confidence, it is much less likely that he or she will take their medical advice. It is important to feel completely comfortable with your doctor and the treatment you get, both on a medical level and a personal level. To that end, it pays to do as much research as you can to ensure that you find the right match. The research should be done ideally, before you get sick, in order to find a doctor and establish a relationship while you are in good health. The following chapter will provide a road map to finding the right practitioner for you.

Know Your Health Plan Restrictions

For those with health insurance, the first step is to know whether the individual practitioner and/or the service needed is covered by your insurance plan. To do so, dust off your health insurance manual – it will have a name, like Certificate of Coverage or Summary of Benefits – or go to your health plan's website and check under "Benefits." See if the kind of practitioner you want is listed under the "Covered Benefits" section and not the "Exclusions" section. Services like chiropractic, acupuncture, or nutrition counseling may or may not be covered benefits, and it is better to know before you incur the expense. If in doubt, most plans have an 800 number for questions.

Next, see whether your health plan tries to direct you to use certain doctors. Health plans have agreements with certain doctors to provide services to their members. These doctors are considered in-network. If you see a doctor who is in-network, the health plan will pay the majority or all of the doctor's charges. However, if you want to see a doctor who is not plan-approved or out-of-network, you pay a higher percentage of that doctor's charges. Always check the terms of your insurance coverage to find out whether your plan will cover visits to the physician you are considering. If he or she does not participate in your health plan, how much will you pay out of pocket for visits to this provider? If you are new to your job and are deciding among different employer-based health plans, you may want to choose a doctor first and then choose the health plan that covers visits to that physician.

Get Recommendations

Start with coworkers, neighbors, and friends. Getting a word-of-mouth referral for a doctor allows you also ask the person why they recommend the doctor and decide if these reasons are important to you. In a recent consumer reports survey, people who found their physicians through someone they trusted – a friend, a family member, or another doctor – had the most favorable experiences.

Options outside of friendly recommendations include cross-checking your health plan's list of doctors with a list of top doctors list in your area. These lists are published in regional magazines like *New York* and *New Jersey Monthly* or the *Washingtonian* and are usually generated by surveying physicians. There are also consumer-ratings websites, like Angie's List or Checkbook, where, for a fee, you can see how other consumers have rated a doctor you may want to visit.

Know the Doctor's Qualifications

So beyond opinion, how do we know whether a particular doctor actually provides a high quality of care? There are a variety of possible sources to check. The most basic question to check off is, "Is this doctor in good professional standing?" Every doctor must be licensed through the state where they practice. The website of the Federation of State Medical Boards (FSMB) has collected data on physicians for more than forty years and provides to the public the FSMB DocInfo Profile. This profile provides professional information on medical doctors, osteopathic physicians, and the majority of physician assistants licensed in the United States. For a fee, the FSMB will provide an instant online answer about prior disciplinary sanctions against a doctor, their educational background, all state licenses held, medical specialty, and their practice location.

A clean FSMB report only ensures that the doctor has never been disciplined for wrongdoing and is licensed to do what they claim to do. The next screening test is to see if a doctor is board certified, but board certification only applies to osteopathic and medical doctors. Board certification involves passing a rigorous exam in a specialty like surgery or family medicine and indicates that the doctor has mastered the body of information for his specialty. You can check on board certification status with the American Board of Medical Specialties, the organization that oversees twenty-four specialty boards, and at websites like HealthGrades and Docfinder.

These initial steps ensure that the doctor is in good standing professionally. Good professional standing is just the minimal expectation you should have for your doctor. What tells you about the way the doctor practices and quality of the care they provide? A few organizations like the National Committee on Quality Assurance (NCQA) have started to recognize doctors based upon whether the individuals they care for are getting good quality care for certain conditions. NCQA-recognized clinicians have met the highest standards of quality care in the areas of heart care, stroke care, diabetes care, and back-pain care using standards agreed upon by recognized experts called quality measures. In addition, the NCQA's Patient-Centered Medical Home (PCMH) is an innovative program for improving primary care. The PCMH is model for providing health care that emphasizes partnerships between individuals, their doctors, and when appropriate, their families; using up-to-date information and communication systems to enhance care provided both during visits and between visits; and making care available to individuals when and where they need and want it. NCQA publishes on their website those primary-care practices – pediatricians, internists, and family medicine physicians – that meet the criteria for excellence in the PCMH model of care. This information is free to the public and accessible at *www.ncqa.org*. In addition, health plans use this data to offer their members networks of high-performing or honor-roll physicians from which they can choose.

> **New with Healthcare Reform:**
> The Physician Compare Initiative started as a result of healthcare reform. It is a government sponsored project, found at Medicare.gov, that includes information on doctor's performances based on quality measures and patient ratings. For no fee, you will be able to look up individual doctors in the Medicare database to get an idea of how they rate.

Finally, if you're picking a doctor to care for a specific condition, it would be great to know how often he or she treats cases similar to yours. While there are no organizations yet that have this information readily available to the public, it is a reasonable question to ask the doctor or their staff over the phone or at your first visit.

Know and Prioritize Your Personal Concerns

Finally, you may have additional concerns when choosing a physician that relate to your own needs and priorities. The first checklist below should help you identify and define further what is most important for you when it comes to the convenience of seeing a doctor. It may be rare for one practitioner to have everything on the list, but you can rank what is a priority for you.

- Location: Is the practice located somewhere it is easy and safe for me to travel? Is there ample parking?

- Hospital Affiliation: Which hospital(s) does the doctor use? Am I comfortable with going for treatment there?

- Testing: Do they have in-office capability for routine X-rays and laboratory studies? If not, how far is the outside laboratory or radiology facility?

- Access to the Doctor: How long do I have to wait for a requested appointment? Are there same-day or walk-in appointments if I have an urgent need? Are the practice hours convenient to my schedule? Are office waits reasonable? If I call or e-mail with a question about my care, does a doctor or nurse answer promptly? Who covers for the physician when he/she is away? Whom should you call if you have a problem after hours? If the doctor works in a group, are you comfortable with being seen by one of the practice partners? (Some experts say that group practices tend to be more efficient and that doctors in groups are more likely to stay up to date on current medical practice.)

- Office Environment: Is the office staff friendly and courteous? Is the waiting room loud or uncomfortable, or is it user friendly?

- Information Access: Does the doctor use electronic records? Does the office have online conveniences like a patient portal for online appointment scheduling, e-mail, providing you lab results and other secure communications?

- Payment: Does the office process insurance claims, or must you pay up front for services and file the claims yourself?

A colleague's elderly mother had a variety of medical problems – arthritis, borderline diabetes, high blood pressure, and chronically poor circulation in her legs. She had an internal medicine doctor, but she and her family felt the doctor was not adequately addressing their concerns. Given the intermittent flare-ups she had with her conditions, she and her family did not have a sense of when to go to the emergency room, go to an urgent care, or try to get an urgent doctor's appointment. The family felt she was slowly getting worse but could not get the responses to the questions they needed answered from her doctor. I encouraged them to go to a geriatrician – one who had experience with care of older adults, their medical problems, and addressing caregiver concerns. This doctor had a reputation of being proactive with her patients. After the first two visits, the family had a clear understanding of her condition, what the warning signs were that signaled her condition was worsening, and how to react to them. She had consultations set up with a nutritionist and an occupational therapist. The doctor also took questions by e-mail, so she and her family felt comfortable that their questions would get answered as needed.

The other major set of concerns relating to choosing a doctor relate to their personal and professional style and character and whether they are a fit for you. This is sometimes a little harder to gauge. You can ask others who have been treated by them or even their office staff. Some physicians are posting video clips of themselves on the HealthGrades website, and for a fee, you can get a feel for their personal style. Nothing replaces meeting the doctor, though, if this is an option. Pediatricians, especially, may be open to an interview appointment to discuss your concerns. You may have to pay a *copayment* or other fee for this service, but it can be a valuable way to gather information when making your decision. When I was helping my mom to choose a doctor when she relocated, we had a bad experience at the first physician we went to because he only talked to me as another physician and not her. So in the interview with the next physician, she was looking specifically for a doctor who would talk to her about her priorities, be respectful, and dialogue directly with her. The goal of the interview with the doctor is to get a feel for their style and how they relate to you. As you talk with them, it may be helpful to evaluate them on the following:

1. Listening skills: Do they let you finish speaking, or do they cut you off? Ask them to state your most important concerns back to you.

2. Attention Span: Do you feel hurried during the encounter? Does the provider give you their full attention, or are there numerous interruptions? If there are interruptions, how do they deal with them? Are they apologetic and respectful of your time?

3. Capacity for compassion: This may be harder to gauge directly. Indirect clues include the following: Does the doctor treat you, other individuals in their practice, and their own staff respectfully? How does the doctor respond to hardships you describe? It would not be out of bounds to even ask the doctor what was their most challenging case and how did they deal with it.

4. Openness to other healing traditions: If this is important to you, be up front if you want to or have tried other

approaches like acupuncture or chiropractic. Your doctor should know about this. See how they respond – are they dismissive, or do they seem open minded, collaborative, or give you specific reasons for including or not including these in your treatment plan in a respectful way?

5. Clarity in explanations and answering questions: Are you able to understand what the doctor is saying? Do they speak in layman's terms using language you can understand? Do they answer your questions directly? Can they provide a clear explanation of what they think is going on? Most importantly, did you leave the office able to explain to someone else what is going on?

6. Promotion of shared decision making: In medicine, for any major decision, there are at least two options – do something or do nothing. Doctors should be able to clearly explain the options and promote you and your priorities in the decision making process. Frequently, under the do-something option, there are several paths that can be taken. The doctor's job is to outline these clearly and help you make the decision that best fits your values. Sometimes, though, because doctors may be hurried, have their own value system, or have a preferred way of doing things, they may not effectively carry this out. One way of assessing your doctor on this is to ask how he involves individuals and their families in decision making.

7. Knowing one's limitations: If the doctor did not know something, how did they deal with this? Did they get defensive or evasive, or did they honestly admit it and seek to get back to you with an answer, or refer to a specialist or someone who could help?

Takeaway Checklist

Finding the provider who is the right fit for you requires asking questions and getting clear answers – both about the doctor and about yourself and what is most important to you.

Doctor Checklist

- ☐ Does your health plan cover the kind of doctor you want, and is the doctor in-network?
- ☐ Seek recommendations through word of mouth, regional publications, and consumer ratings sites.
- ☐ Find the doctor's qualifications, background, and professional standing.
- ☐ Find out the quality of care the doctor provides.

Personal Preference Checklist

- ☐ Location
- ☐ Hospital affiliation
- ☐ In-office testing capability
- ☐ Ease of accessing the doctor
- ☐ Office environment
- ☐ Online presence
- ☐ Form of payment accepted
- ☐ Professional style – ability to listen, be open to other healing traditions, be clearly understood, involve you in decision making, and respond to uncertainty

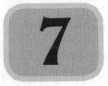

Relating to Your Doctor – How To Be Your Best Advocate

*It is easy to get a thousand prescriptions
but hard to get one single remedy.*

– Chinese Proverb

I have had personal experience with the need to be my own health advocate, yet another experience that influenced me to write this book. In the process of moving into a new home, lifting, twisting, and working above shoulder level, I developed a sore back and neck. I did a series of stretches improperly to try to stretch out my back and neck. Over the next few days, my neck pain worsened to the point where I could not turn my head to the left at all. By the third night of this, it felt like my throat was closing when I lay down, and I could not breathe. My fiancé took me to the emergency department. I told the doctor my symptoms, told him I was an ED doctor also, and that I thought I needed a neck MRI. Because it was 2:00 a.m., the MRI tech was not in, so he said he would do a CT scan instead. He gave me some heavy duty IV pain meds, which made me sleepy, and sent me off to CT. The CT scan, of course, was normal. He discharged me with a prescription for some anti-anxiety pills. I was too drugged up to protest, so I went home to sleep it off. A few hours after I got home, I got a call from the chief of emergency medicine at the hospital where I had been. He had reviewed my chart, saw I was a doctor, what I had said about my breathing and my request for an MRI. He invited me to come back in. The MRI showed I had a torn neck muscle that was bleeding, resulting in a buildup of blood inside my neck. The collection of blood was pushing on my airway, hence the feeling I could not breathe. I had emergency surgery to get the blood out and have since been fine. If I had been a lay person and had not known to ask for the MRI, what would the outcome have been?

NOW THAT YOU have chosen your professional partner in health, it is important to build a successful working relationship with that person. Surveys show that the people most satisfied with their care are those who share the responsibility for their health with their doctors. Your doctor is an expert on medical care, but you are the expert on yourself. Partnering with your doctor will involve choosing the option for treating your condition that best fits your values, beliefs, and lifestyle. If you are not satisfied with your care, it is important to communicate that. If it falls on deaf ears, there are plenty of other doctors to go to for another opinion. Once you find the right doctor, you will feel better about carrying out the chosen treatment that feels right. This chapter will detail how to go about establishing a partnering relationship with your health-care provider at each phase of your journey.

Preparing for the Visit

So by now you have started learning about your condition, started to make lifestyle changes, and researched the type(s) of health-care provider you need. You may have even had an appointment or two. How do you go about getting the most out of each encounter with your doctor or provider?

At each new encounter with a health-care provider, you want to make sure to prepare adequately for the visit. Preparation entails more than bringing your insurance card and ID. It involves having the information the doctor will need to best be able to help you. Addressing the following items before every visit will ensure that the visit is an efficient process where you have your major concerns addressed.

1. What you take: Ensure that you have a list of any medications and their dosages, including vitamins and over-the-counter products like Tylenol, aspirin, or cough syrup. If you do not have a list, just bring the medication containers with you.

2. A health buddy: Remember your support network we discussed? Now it is time to activate it. Take a friend or family member who you trust with you to your visit. A buddy is especially important if your condition is complex, if you are not feeling well or if decisions need to be made, like starting on a new medication or having surgery. Even if you are a very private or independent person, there are several reasons why this is helpful. This additional trusted heath buddy can be an extra set of eyes and ears when you talk to the doctor. They can be writing things down as you do the talking. When you are not feeling well, it is easy to miss the critical information discussed at the visit. This person may also help to understand what the doctor discusses or ask questions that may not occur to you. A health buddy can even play the role of your advocate. There are also organizations that will provide health advocates, or you can hire the services of a medical companion to go to MD visits with you for this purpose.

3. Know your history: It is important to be able to fill in the picture for any practitioner you may be seeing for the first time. List any conditions that you have or take previous records from other doctors. You can request prior health records from any hospital or doctor who treated you. Alternatively, your new doctor can initiate the request with your written permission. Getting your medical records may

involve a fee for making hardcopies or for a digital copy of the record.

There are a number of tools that can help you to keep these important pieces of your health information organized. There are simple written checklists in the form of pamphlets that can be updated at each visit. For the more web savvy, personal health records (PHRs) have the potential to give individuals more control over their health information – collecting, using, and sharing it as they see fit. PHRs are an online record of you and your family's health records. You have access to input and update the information as needed. PHRs use secure technology to protect your information from being seen without permission. You can share the record electronically with your provider's office, carry it with you as a mobile app, or print it out to take a hardcopy. Access to a PHR can be purchased as a subscription or obtained free through your employer, insurance company, or doctor's office. Free PHRs are often maintained by the health-care organization that hosts them and are updated with your latest health information, including diagnosis, medications, lab and test results, each time you have an encounter. Some PHRs let you refill prescriptions, schedule appointments, e-mail your doctor, and learn more about your condition and medications.

During the Encounter

The process through which a doctor arrives at a diagnosis depends heavily upon what you tell them is bothering you. Most conventional doctors spend a limited time, usually ten to fifteen minutes, interacting with each patient. Even for practitioners who can spend more time, it is still important to be prepared to make the most of that time with clear information about your specific concerns. So always start with the main problem or most troubling symptoms first. Be ready to describe the symptoms, when and how they started, their frequency and duration, what makes them better or worse, how they affect your ability to do daily activities, and any past experiences you have had with the same problem.

Questions to Ask During the Visits: This list of questions may not be relevant at every visit, but you can adapt them to the nature of the visit you are having. The answers to the questions should be written down during or immediately after the visit by you or your health buddy. With the doctor's permission, you can even tape the encounter so there is no doubt about the takeaway points for later reference. It is important to update any medical records that you keep with the information you gain.

- **What's wrong?** The answer you get from the practitioner should never be the same symptom that you told the doctor, like knee pain or cough. It should be the doctor's diagnosis that includes an explanation of why you feel like you do. This should be provided to you in simple, layman's terms. Occasionally, doctors are not sure what the problem is immediately and have to order tests. In this case, ask the doctor to tell you the top two or three diagnoses he is trying to eliminate or establish and how the tests will help in this evaluation.
- **What do I need to know about what you are prescribing?** If the doctor orders tests, medications, or

procedure, understand their purpose and how they will help treat you or get to the bottom of your problem. Specifics to ask your doctor about his plans for you include:

- What's the name of the medicine/test/ procedure/ surgery?
- Why do I need it?
- What are the risks or potential side effects? Can it interfere with anything I am taking/eating? Can the procedure/test/medicine injure me in any way?
- Are there other options?
- What is the cost? Is it covered by my insurance?
- What happens if I do nothing or do not take the treatment/test/surgery?

For Tests/Surgery/ Procedures Only:

- How do I prepare for the test/procedure/surgery?

For Medications Only:

- Do you have free samples or coupons to get it at a discount?
- How do I take this medicine?
- Is there a generic version I can take?
- Review you medications regularly with both your doctor and pharmacist to understand the potential side effects. This is especially true if you are on multiple medicines, and a new one is being added. Your doctor should make efforts, whenever possible, to minimize

the number of medicines you are taking. And read the packaging from your pharmacy or medication insert so you can know for yourself what potential side effects are.

- **What do I do going forward?** Frequently, the treatment being prescribed may just be the first step. It is important to be clear about the next steps going forward. The following questions will help you to know what these next steps are:

    - Do I need to return for a follow-up visit? When will it be?
    - When will the results be ready? Can I phone in for test results, or will you call me? How can I get copies of any test results?
    - Are there referrals to specialists? Why is the referral needed?
    - If there are referrals to others like therapists, case managers, or social workers, what is the purpose?

- **What I can do at home?** You and/or your caregiver, after all, will be the ones doing the day-to-day interventions to address your condition. Always ask what you can be doing to improve your health.

    - How should I care for ___? (for example, my ankle sprain, my headaches, my high blood sugar)
    - What behaviors/foods/actions should I avoid?
    - What behaviors/foods/actions should I start?
    - What danger signs should I look for?

- When do I need to report back about my condition?

And just to make sure you covered all the bases, end with "Is there anything else I need to know?" If you are uncomfortable with any of the aspects of treatment or cannot carry them out, let the doctor know and make sure to explore any alternatives that you can follow through on.

Getting a Second Opinion

Most Americans trust their doctors and do not feel the need to seek out a second opinion, according to a 2010 Gallup poll. The poll also showed that older Americans tended to be more trusting of their doctors, although there was no difference in trust level related to educational achievement or gender.

On the other hand, studies show that patients get the wrong diagnosis as much as 20 percent of the time, and the wrong treatment half of the time. There are many reasons for a misdiagnosis, and it is not always related to the competency of the doctor or because they did not spend as much time per patient visit as they once could. Sometimes it may be too early in the course of the illness to diagnosis it correctly. Other times, it has to do with the complexity of the problem, which ends up requiring multiple doctors who might not be easily available, especially in rural or underrepresented urban communities. For example, a University of Michigan study showed that when women who already had a treatment plan for their breast cancer were seen by a panel of health providers from different specialties, the interpretation of the mammogram and recommendation for surgery was changed in more than half the patients (77/149 or 52 percent). That is because treatment of breast cancers, as with many other cancers, are ideally done by doctors from several disciplines, including surgeons, oncologists, radiologists, pathologists, radiation oncologists, and nurses. This approach is already the standard of care in most major cancer centers in the United States, which might not be seen in areas where cancer centers are not available.

So where does this leave someone with a new or rare diagnosis? Oftentimes, individuals are reluctant to seek help outside of their established doctor because they feel like (1) they are betraying the relationship, or (2) if their doctor finds out, they will be mad at them and not continue to give them the best care. However, when faced with a new diagnosis or worsening of your condition despite treatment, going to another doctor for a second or even third opinion is not betraying your first doctor. This is about your well-being and overall health and not about the doctor's ego or even your relationship with him. No good doctor ever dropped a patient for getting another opinion, and some may even help by referring you to other doctor's they respect. I helped a patient with a rare condition, optic neuritis, to find a second opinion on what was causing it. His first ophthalmologist was not able to help. We were able to find a neuro-ophthalmologist in a large center who had treated numerous cases. He correctly diagnosed the condition, explained what it was, and started the patient on the effective treatment right away. When faced with a rare or complex condition, going to centers where they are commonly treated, even if it means travel, is a good approach.

How do you find these centers of excellence? The first good person to ask is your doctor. If you do not want to do this or do not yet have a doctor, there are several other reliable resources. You can check with foundations and organizations who may be dedicated to education and fundraising to find a cure for your condition. Organizations like those for diabetes, heart disease, and rheumatoid arthritis offer advice about what centers and doctors are considered the experts on the condition and which ones are closest to your area. More obscure diseases also have dedicated advocacy groups that provide information on their website. Another option is asking other individuals with your condition who have been treated successfully. There are a number of support groups on the Internet that provide discussion groups where you can meet others with your condition and compare notes.

Tracking Your Progress

When working on your health with a health-care professional as your partner, it is crucial to be able to track your progress. The very first step is to know what your goal is. Studies show that people who have a goal and are clear about it try harder, are more focused on the change, and are more likely to stick with what is required to achieve it. In short, people with goals are often the people who succeed. To this end, you should have a frank discussion with your doctor to define your treatment goals and know exactly what specific self-health actions are required of you to reach them. For a goal to work, you need a clear plan to support it. One time tested way of doing this is to take the self-health actions expected of you and create SMART goals. That is, they should be:

SPECIFIC: Your goals should be clear and precise. For example, instead of "get healthy," specify "lower my blood pressure to 120/80."

MEASURABLE: You must be able to measure your progress toward meeting your goals. For example, instead of "start walking," make it "walk one mile four days a week."

ACTION-ORIENTED: Your goals should include action-oriented behavior that is totally in your control.

REALISTIC: Set a goal that is within your reach. For example, realistic weight loss is 1-2 lbs a week.

TIMED: Set a time frame within which to evaluate your progress or meet your goals. This could be a time frame, like two weeks, or a specific date.

And then you need to track your progress toward it. One possible advantage of tracking is that it generates a feeling of satisfaction that further motivates you to work harder to reach your targets. Another advantage is to know if you are on the right path. Your doctor should let you know what tests he or she is using to monitor your progress and how often it is being tracked. Finally, as you achieve your goals, do not forget to celebrate even a seemingly small victory.

Another point to be absolutely clear about with your treatment plan is what the signs of success, or failure, are along the way. Your doctor should review these with you. For example, if you have type 2 diabetes, success may look like getting your hemoglobin A1C down to 7 percent. If you are being treated for breast cancer, it may be taking your anti-vomiting medicine every 8 hours so you can drink liquids and stay well hydrated while receiving chemotherapy.

Some treatments, like acupuncture for certain conditions, may result in your condition getting temporarily worse before it gets better. You should know if temporary worsening is a sign of success and how long this period should last before you get better or get concerned. Other treatments may take weeks instead of hours or days to have an effect, like medical treatments for nerve pain, and you should know not to give up before your goal is reached.

Communication Breakdowns: One of the most frequent doctor-patient communication problems I see is when treatments do not initially work. Instead of getting back to the doctor to let them know, individuals write off their doctors and may go to ERs and urgent cares, unsuccessfully looking for a quick fix. One individual who consulted me had a recurring rash and a cluster of other concerning symptoms for several weeks. He had been to his primary doctor early on before the full manifestation of the condition occurred. His doctor told him it was a viral illness and prescribed accordingly. When other symptoms cropped up, instead of going back to the doctor, he went to an urgent care and the next week an ER. In doing so, his primary doctor, who had seen him in the beginning, got cut out of the picture and was significantly delayed in making the real diagnosis of lupus, which was not apparent until more symptoms showed themselves. I was able to help breach the gap and found that the communication breakdown was two-way – the doctor did not make it clear to call him back if symptoms changed and the patient did not call back and say, "Hey, things are not going well. You need to see me again." On the other hand, a patient suffering seasonal allergies went to see a homeopathic pharmacist, who clearly stated, "If this does not work in three days, come back and see me." The patient felt confident that there was an open-door policy and a clear partnership in getting a fix to her symptoms.

On the flip side, you should also know what it looks like if your treatment or your plan is not working. Warning signs are those symptoms which signal to you that things are going in the wrong direction. You should have a list of these symptoms that are specific to your condition – such as shortness of breath if you have asthma. It is also important to know those warning signs that relate to the treatments you are receiving – like heartburn, if you are taking a medicine like Fosamax for osteoporosis or if you develop a fever after a procedure. You should also have an action plan for warning signs since some are potentially more serious than others. Review these with your doctor, and know which ones require urgent attention and which ones can be reported to your doctor at your next visit.

Tracking your symptoms to know if the treatment is working or not and providing this feedback to your health-care provider is a key part of your treatment. Observations about how you are responding to treatment are key pieces of information only you and your caregiver can provide. To that end, it is helpful to have a symptom diary in which you record treatment dose and time, daily symptoms you experience before and after your treatment, and how your symptoms vary from day to day or progress week over week.

If your symptoms persist longer than what your doctor has outlined, your doctor should review your current treatment plan and your overall health to be sure nothing was missed. If you have not followed your treatment plan, it is important to be up front with your doctor and discuss the pitfalls you are experiencing. Together with your doctor, you can figure out ways that will improve your ability to successfully follow the plan, including modifying the plan if necessary. If you feel your doctor is not responding to a lack of success with the treatment plan despite your sticking with it, that is exactly the time to seek a second opinion.

Takeaway Checklist

A successful working relationship with your provider is one where you share responsibility with them for your health. This checklist helps you to prepare to take a proactive role when interacting with your health-care professional

- ☐ Prepare for each visit by knowing your health history and having a list of any medications you take – online tools can help you stay organized.
- ☐ Activate your support network, and bring a health buddy to your visit.
- ☐ Ask questions at your visit, so when you leave you can explain to someone else what is going on with you and your treatment plan.

  - o What is wrong with me?
  - o What do I need to know about the treatment and its effects, side effects, and cost?
  - o What are the alternatives to taking the prescribed treatment?
  - o What are the next steps?
  - o What self-care actions do I need to do at home?

- ☐ Get a second opinion if you are not comfortable with your diagnosis.

☐ Track your progress

    o   Know your treatment goals and set SMART goals based on them.

    o   Know how to figure out whether the treatment plan is working – the signs of success and the warning signs that the treatment is not working.

    o   Keeping a symptom diary will make it easier to convey to the doctor how you are responding.

☐ Get a second opinion if your doctor does not respond to a lack of progress despite your communicating with him and sticking to the treatment plan. Centers of excellence are good options to find other doctors for second opinions.

Your Hospital Stay – Thriving Through It and Beyond

*In Turkey, you're not allowed to be left
alone in the hospital. The nurse teaches
the family how to do things, and somebody
is always there with the patient.*

– Dr. Mehmet Oz

So now we have covered choosing and forming an effective working relationship with a professional partner in health. But we have only covered care you may receive in an office setting. What if you have an illness which requires a hospital stay? What should you know about hospital care and specifically how to get the best care when in the hospital?

One of my motivations for writing this book, and this chapter especially, was an experience my family had when trying to get treatment for my dad, who had Parkinson's disease. He was pretty debilitated when he went into the hospital. My family and I went to great lengths to find a hospital where there was expertise in the care of Parkinson's disease. Beforehand, and again on the day he was admitted, I had lengthy discussions with the doctor who supervised his care. I explained that he was on an every-other-day dose of his blood pressure medication. His dose had decreased over time because of his weight loss from the Parkinson's, and his blood pressure had naturally been coming down. I also explained that he might not even need blood pressure medications at all, given his present state. She assured me they would minimize the dose, and I felt reassured he was in good hands. So imagine my shock when I came in the next morning, only to find them trying to resuscitate my dad due to a loss of blood pressure! It turns out that not only did they give him blood pressure medicine, they also gave him a higher dose than he was on before getting to the hospital. What had happened? The attending doctor had not conveyed to the junior doctors – the resident who wrote the orders – our conversation. The resident just saw "high blood pressure" on the chart, wrote for a standard dose of blood pressure medicine, and called it a day. My father survived this incident as well as others that were not as life threatening. But it really opened my eyes to that fact that if I, as a physician, could not rely on a vigilant hospital staff, how did the family of a lay person, who was not medically trained, make it out of the hospital uneventfully?

MANY PEOPLE DO not make it out of the hospital uneventfully. It has been ten years since the Institute of Medicine estimated that medical errors cause up to ninety-eight thousand deaths in hospitals each year, and still almost one in four hospitalized individuals continue to be harmed during their stays. In addition, because the handoff of care is sometimes not done well when people leave the hospital to go to a nursing facility or back home, about 20 percent of discharged seniors are ending up right back in hospital within thirty days. The fact of the matter is that choosing a place to get health care is more than just finding the best doctor and going to the hospital where they practice. In going to a hospital, we are choosing a whole team of individuals – from the floor secretary, to the X-ray technician, to the cleaning staff, to the transportation aides – and a system of care that will shape our experience. Oftentimes, the patients' complaints and the medical errors made are related to the lack of one person who is responsible for the quality of the entire experience. Care, even within a hospital, can be fragmented and disjointed with poor communication between the various team members and even among the doctors themselves. So what can you do to advocate for the best quality hospital care for yourself?

Choose a High-Quality Hospital

Worldwide, America has the highest cost of medical care. So that equates to the highest quality of health care in the world, right? Well, not exactly. Though we lead in innovation and have some of the most highly trained doctors and advanced treatments, high quality of care is not found uniformly throughout our health-care system. We tend to pick our doctors and hospitals for convenience rather than any specific criteria related to how well they give care. This is very different from how we make the rest of the major spending decisions in our lives – researching, looking for deals, and evaluating quality.

One big reason for our selection decisions was the lack of information available to the public about hospital quality. There was no public information source detailing how well hospitals were doing in caring for customers – making sure they were leaving in better condition than when they came in, or that they did not have to immediately return to the hospital after going home. However, thanks to health-care reform, the federal government is now keeping track. Hospitals are now required to report how well they perform on certain quality measures. In turn, the Department of Health and Human Services organizes this information and publishes it for easy public access. Hospital quality rankings are based upon a variety of criteria that can be grouped as follows:

a. **How efficiently the hospital provides standard treatments for certain common conditions** – these measures tell how often or how quickly a hospital is giving the appropriate treatments for common conditions like heart attack and pneumonia. Examples include how quickly a clot-busting medicine that restores blood flow to the heart is given for heart attacks, or how often people with pneumonia get the right antibiotic medicine.

b. **Complication rates from common procedures** – these statistics indicate how well individuals do after common surgeries, like a hip replacement, and how effective hospitals are at avoiding complications after surgery, such as infection or blood clots.

c. **Survival rates from common illnesses** – these statistics are an indirect measure of how well hospitals are taking care of people with common ailments like pneumonia and heart attacks. Some hospitals take care of sicker patients than others, so their survival statistics may look worse. However, the numbers are adjusted to account for these differences so that hospitals can be compared fairly.

d. **Readmission rates** – readmission rates measure how many patients return for admission within thirty days. Rates of readmission show whether a hospital is doing its best to ensure those leaving make a smooth transition to home or another setting such as a nursing home. Coordinating a smooth transition out of the hospital includes ensuring that the person is physically well enough to be discharged; checking that new medicines and medicines prior to the hospitalization do not conflict with each other; educating individuals about their condition, including diet restrictions, physical restrictions, and all medications; creating a post hospital care plan that is well coordinated among all those involved – the family or caregiver, rehab facility, home health agency, or doctor's office; and ensuring all medical supplies and equipment will be delivered to the home in time for the patient's arrival. While readmissions data is collected for only three conditions – stroke, heart attack, and pneumonia – it can serve as an indicator of how closely the hospital is paying attention to these details for all conditions, including yours.

e. **Patient satisfaction** – experiences of other consumers can help you judge how tuned in the hospital is to the priorities of its clients and their families – items like comfort, noise level, communication, respect, emotional support, continuity of care, and involvement of family and friends.

f. **Medical imaging rates** – most common radiology imaging procedures, like CAT scans and X-rays, use radiation. Overuse of radiation can promote the formation of certain cancers. Some estimates predict that 2 percent of all future cancers will result from the increasing use of imaging. Because of the risks of radiation, an important measure of quality of care is the number of unnecessary CT scans performed for conditions like back pain and sinus disease. Rushing straight to an imaging study is rarely necessary because it bypasses simpler, safer, and effective methods of diagnosis and treatment. These quality measures show how often doctors and hospitals order CT scans and other radiology studies only when absolutely needed.

While there are a number of hospital-quality comparison websites, the five below are easy to use and present hospital quality indicators in ways consumers can use. The bottom line is you want to use this information to make an informed decision about the safest hospitals that you can access.

Medicare Quality Care Finder *http://www.medicare.gov/ quality-care-finder/* – this federally administered website provides quality rankings not just for hospitals, but also doctors, nursing homes, home health agencies, dialysis facilities, and drug and health plans. Their rankings are based on a possible five-star rating system. For hospitals specifically, the section of the website is called HospitalCompare. There you can compare the quality of care at hospitals in your area and across the country. You can get hospital contact information, patient survey results, rates of readmission, mortality (death) rates, and more.

Report Cards for Hospitals in New York, California, Texas, Washington, and Florida from MyHealthFinder.com, and for Ohio, on *http://ohiohospitalcompare.ohio.gov*. These sites show how hospitals within a state compare to each other. They also include multiple measures of patient's satisfaction and safety.

Health Grades.com is a health-care quality ratings site that rates both doctors and hospitals. Hospitals are rated by certain measures so, for example, you can find out how a hospital compares on rates of complications for common procedures like hip replacement or prostate removal. You can also see the survival rates for common illnesses like pneumonia, stroke, and heart attack.

US News and Health Reports publishes a yearly ranking of large academic hospitals based on a combination of government data and surveys of hospitals, health-care consumers, and medical experts. The hospital must offer at least four of eight specific medical technologies, such as a PET/CT scanner and certain radiation therapies. They are ranked based on reputation, patient survival, patient safety, and care-related factors such as nursing and patient services.

The Commonwealth Fund at *http://whynotthebest.org/* – this website allows you to compare overall recommended care, surgical care, and care for pneumonia, heart failure, and heart attacks against other hospitals in a geographic area.

Be Hospital-Wise

Even after you have done your research and found a well-rated hospital, it is still important to be mindful about the care you get when you enter the hospital. There are four key principles that should govern how you approach the experience. These are the following:

1. Be the missing link.
2. The squeaky wheel gets the most oil.
3. Maximize the strength and protection of your fortress.
4. Bring an advocate.

Each of these principles will stand you in good stead as you go through your hospital experience. Let us explore each one in more detail.

1. **Be the missing link** – poor communication between health-care providers in the hospital setting is one of the leading causes of medical errors. You may be the missing link for facilitating communication between the various people who come in contact with you and impact your care.
   a. To that end, it is important to come to the hospital prepared with an accurate and updated list of all your

current medications, allergies, and dietary restrictions. It is best to have several written copies to make available to anyone who asks and therefore not have to rely on memory to ensure you answer questions correctly and are given the right medications.

b. Another part of being the missing link is to know the game plan, especially if several doctors are involved with your care. Knowing the game plan involves knowing your treatment plan and procedures that are planned. If there are any inconsistencies or deviations, insist on a prompt and thorough explanation and keep asking until you get a satisfactory answer. The game plan also involves knowing all of the medications you are prescribed once admitted to the hospital – their names, dosages, and purposes. You should double-check to be sure that you are being given the correct medications in the correct dosages and at the proper interval.

c. Keep a notepad by the bed to write down all your questions in preparation for your doctor's once-a-day visit to see you. Any unanswered questions will have to wait until the following day; or you may have to ask the nurse to call the doctor for the answer which may or may not be successful.

d. When the doctor does come, ask if you can record the conversation on your cell phone or tape recorder. That way, you can listen later to make sure you catch and understand everything that was said and also share it with other caregivers who may not be there at the time.

e. Finally, insist on double-checking of labels. This will help to avoid patient, record, drug, and procedure mix-ups, which do occasionally happen. You can ask staff to refer to you by name, look at the label on the drug itself, and make sure labels are correct, including which body part will have surgery.

2. **The squeaky wheel gets the most oil** – just as the squeaky wheel gets the most oil, being vocal about your needs will ensure you get the required attention. Unfortunately, hospital staff are pulled in a thousand different directions. They can easily overlook or make a lower priority the individual and their family who is quiet and makes no requests. At the same time, be nice and not demanding, because you do not want to be the person whom the staff avoids. Some sample scenarios of you or your caregiver being a squeaky wheel in the hospital setting include the following:

a. Alerting the nurse or doctor immediately if something seems wrong or you or your loved one is in pain or discomfort – continue to remind staff until it is addressed.

b. When in doubt about making a decision, saying no and requiring an explanation until you understand the issue and feel comfortable you have the information you need.

c. Asking for a copy of all test results and requesting explanations of their meaning. It is easy to assume that no news means everything is OK, but it may also mean something fell through the cracks. If something seems wrong, request a repeat.

d. It is OK to change your team: If you do not feel that a doctor or staff member is competent, caring, or providing the proper care, politely but firmly insist that they be removed from your health-care team.

3. **Maximize the strength and protection of your fortress** – isn't it ironic that when people are at their weakest and most vulnerable to illness, they are put in a place where there are the most germs? Hospitals can be a downright dirty place, full of bacteria and viruses that can wreak havoc on your body when your immune system is low. However, there are some steps you can take to minimize the chances of getting hospital-related infections.

a. Keep germs away whenever possible by boldly asking whoever is going to touch you, family and health-care workers, to make sure they wash their hands first. That includes also asking doctors to wipe their stethoscope with an alcohol pad. Stethoscopes are carriers of germs because often, doctors forget to clean them between exams. Keep your own hands clean as much as possible and avoid letting visitors sit on your bed. Ask your doctors and nurses each day about when IVs, urinary catheters, and any other tubes in your body can come out since risk of infection grows the longer they stay in. Finally, rooms should be cleaned daily with special attention to surfaces that harbor germs like bed rails, bedside tables, IV poles, call bells, door handles, bathroom surfaces, and computer keyboards. Environmental services (ES) staff should put on a new pair of gloves when they enter your room, and if you believe they have missed something, kindly point it out to them.

b. Keep your body primed for recovery and to fight infections. This is most achievable when you are going into the hospital for an elective procedure and have time to prepare. If you are overweight or obese, aim to lose 10 percent of your body weight and strengthen your muscles prior to the procedure – it will shorten your recovery time and lessen the possibility of complications. This is especially true for abdominal and pelvic surgeries like hysterectomies, gallbladder removals, and hernia repairs. Muscle strengthening is especially key for bone and joint surgeries like knee replacements, and your doctor can prescribe physical therapy eight weeks prior to the operation solely for this purpose. Finally, well-nourished individuals respond to and recover from illness and surgery better than those who are undernourished. So if you know you will be having a future procedure, refer back to the "Self-Health Actions" described before to best prepare your body for it.

c. Avoid unnecessary medicines that may lower your body's defenses – one of these medicines is a heartburn drug known as a proton pump inhibitor (PPI) used to prevent stress-related heartburn while in the hospital. However, because PPIs neutralize the same stomach acid which protects us against bacterial invaders, they can make you more likely to get intestinal infections and pneumonias. If you are not being treated for severe heartburn or ulcers, you should discuss with your doctor whether you need them or not.

4. **Bring an Advocate** – having your own advocate is the key to carrying out steps one through three. If you are sick, it is too much to keep up with all of this by yourself. Your main job is getting better. Have the best communicator or most persistent, detailed-oriented person you know – friend or family – take notes and talk with health personnel about your case. Your advocate is one who learns the treatment plan, asks questions, double-checks, and speaks up. Doctors and staff are forced to pay more attention to you and to details of your case when someone else is around, being your eyes, ears, and voice. If no one exists like this for you, some hospitals now have patient navigator programs or private patient advocate services to assist you while in the hospital.

Another role for your advocate is that of gatekeeper for you. While it is important to keep in touch, it is equally important to limit contact with well-meaning friends and family so that you can rest and recover. There are websites, like *www. caringbridge.org*, that allow people to connect, communicate, and get updated information on hospitalized loved ones. You or your advocate can post information, maintain a diary, and allow people password access to stay updated on your condition and communicate with you.

There is a silver lining to hospital care. There are trends brought about by health-care reform which may be improving the care you get in the hospital. Because it takes money, time, and resources to change the way business is done, hospitals have had no monetary incentive to improve the way they provide care. Until now. Because of health-care reform, hospitals will get financial incentives for improving patient care from public insurance payers like Medicare and private ones like Aetna or United. Conversely, they stand to lose thousands of dollars for failing to improve on quality of care since someone is actually paying attention and keeping track now. As a result, hospitals are trying to improve the care they provide. In the near future, this should translate to better communication between hospital staff, better communication with the consumers, and better processes to ensure hospital errors are minimized at every turn.

Leaving the Hospital

Leaving the hospital is a big achievement because that usually means you are doing better and require less intensive care than you did before. But how carefully you prepare for departure is just as important as the care you got in the hospital. Hospitals call this process "discharge planning." Paying attention to all the steps involved can determine how successful you are at not having to come right back into the hospital. Attention to details can aid with continuing a smooth recovery outside the hospital and reduce stress for those helping to care for you. Planning for the transition out of the hospital is important no matter what your destination is once you leave the hospital – your own home, a friend or family member's house, or to a rehabilitation center or nursing home.

The Discharge Planning Process

Discharge planners are staff in the hospital whose main job is to work with families to help plan the transition out of the hospital and help arrange for continued care. The discharge planners focus on:

1. whether it is possible to safely return to your original living situation;
2. training for those who will be caregivers – this includes providing them with a written summary of the hospital stay, a list of medications, potential warning signs of a worsening condition, and contact information in case of questions or concerns;
3. whether third-party care is needed, such as a skilled nursing facility, rehab facility, or home care service, and what the most appropriate location is, considering your health status, where you live, and religious, language, and/or cultural issues; and
4. whether any extra equipment, such as wheelchairs or breathing assistance devices, will be necessary in the new setting.

So what are some of the things you and your family can do to make sure this process goes well? Fortunately, the checklist of actions is similar whether you are going to a home environment or a nursing facility. Another hallmark of good discharge planning is that it starts at the beginning of the hospital admission. To that end, the checklist of action items for you and your family starts during the hospital stay and continues up until the time of discharge.

During the Hospital Stay:

- Start recording the names and roles of all the doctors involved in treatment during the hospital stay and how best to contact them post discharge if you have questions later.

- Request a physical and occupational therapy evaluation prior to leaving the hospital. Most hospitals will do this automatically if your condition is complex, has left you weakened, or you have had a long hospital stay. These evaluations will reveal how much you are able to function, including providing an idea of how long it may take to show improvement. This step is also essential to determine what setting will be best for you to continue your recovery after discharge, and how much help will be needed during the recovery period.

- Touch bases with your health insurer to find out about the services and coverage available post hospitalization. Do they have a case manager that will help with coordinating discharge planning? Do they cover home health services and for how long? The same questions should be asked for coverage of skilled nursing facilities – most health plans have limits of thirty days, and have in-network contracts with certain facilities to allow for lower out-of-pocket costs. The hospital discharge planner and insurance company case manager should be able to help identify those facilities that are in-network.

- Both the rehabilitation evaluations and the discharge planner should provide guidance on where you should stay after being discharged. If it is in the home setting, decisions need to be made about who will help with continued care, medical care, as well as daily tasks, and if changes need to be made to the home to accommodate your needs.

Just Prior to Leaving the Hospital:

- Get a written list of all tests, procedures, and treatments that were done, and any available as well as pending results; and any follow-up treatments or procedures that need to be scheduled.

- Review your medication(s) with the doctor or nurse prior to leaving the hospital. This includes dosage, number of times to be taken per day, and whether it is to be administered with or without food. This review should also reconcile any new medicines started with ones that you were already taking prior to going into the hospital. Find out if there is a twenty-four-hour service number for questions dealing with medications, dosage, interactions, and complications.

- Make sure there is a follow-up appointment scheduled within ten days with your personal physician and any other physicians involved in the hospital care. This step is *essential* to make sure that the adjustment to the transition out of the hospital is going well and that the treatment plan is proceeding as intended.

- Have a list of the medical supplies you may need if going home and have the corresponding prescriptions.

- You/your caregiver should get training to know warning signs of potential problems, including when to call the doctor or go to the ER. Training should also cover nutritional needs; foods to avoid; if needed, how to move and care for you; wound care; and any medical treatment that needs to be provided after leaving the hospital. This is especially important if medical equipment, like glucose meters, breathing machines, or heart monitors, is needed. Get a direct telephone number for issues or concerns relating to any equipment.

• Ask for a list of support groups that specialize in your illness as well as any organizations that provide counseling for the needs of caregivers. We will cover caregiver needs later in this chapter.

Choosing a Nursing Home or Rehabilitation Facility

Some individuals may be faced with the need to choose a rehabilitation or skilled nursing facility, also called a nursing home. Choosing a high-quality facility is important to ensure you or your loved one is getting the right care in a time where they may be the most fragile. As an emergency doctor, one of the most frustrating parts of my job was caring for individuals who came from skilled nursing facilities. The most common reasons why emergency evaluation was needed were often entirely preventable. Frequent turning in bed can prevent skin breakdown and subsequent infection. Regular changing of bladder catheters or IV lines can prevent severe skin, urine, or blood infections. Close monitoring of medication doses and nutritional intake can avoid confusion, bleeding, and dehydration. Paying attention to quality of care issues such as these at the facility you are considering can be the difference between a smooth recovery or poor care and a return to the hospital.

Again, thanks to health-care reform, many institutions are now being more closely monitored and have financial incentives to provide a higher quality of care. As with hospitals, there are resources now available for consumers to help identify facilities to avoid. Working with the hospital discharge planner and the insurance case manager, there are often more choices in rehabilitation or skilled nursing facilities than in hospitals. The hospital where you end up may be the choice of the ambulance driver in an emergency; but for the rehabilitation or skilled nursing facility, there is usually more time to research the options. Insurance companies also only include those facilities in their network that provide higher quality care – it would not be in their financial interest to contract with providers who cause complications and multiple hospitalizations. So it is sometimes better to choose a facility that your insurance company has contracted with since you pay less out of pocket, and they have often been prescreened.

Medicare.gov under *Quality Care Finder (http://www.medicare. gov/quality-care-finder/)* is also a source of information about nursing facilities. At the Medicare website, you can see health inspector reports, the staffing ratio, and the quality of care being provided – like how often residents get pressure sores or urine infections – and whether the facility has been cited and had to pay fines in the past. The website also shows those facilities that have been cited for problems and if these problems were remedied.

Once you have narrowed it down to two or three possibilities, there are some additional questions you should ask of the facility and the hospital discharge planner. If possible, a visit to the prospective facility by your family or caregiver could yield additional information and provide an opportunity to observe and also speak with the staff, residents, and residents' families to get a sense of the following:

- Why was this type of facility suggested?
- What specific medical needs does this facility address?
- Can this facility meet all your needs, or will additional assistance be necessary?
- How close and convenient is this facility for the family and caregiver to visit?
- Is it clean, quiet, and comfortable?
- Does this facility address any nutritional, cultural, or language-related issues specific to you or your loved one?
- What is the staff to resident ratio?
- Do residents get the assistance they need in a timely fashion?
- Does the staff listen attentively and respectfully to residents?
- Does the atmosphere appear homelike, or is it institutional?

Choosing a Home Health-Care Service

If your needs are not extensive enough to require facility care, you can receive care in a home setting from family or friends. Home health agencies can be a big part of providing the care needed with both medical and nonmedical services.

There are two different kinds of home health agencies. The first kind of home health agency provides medical services, similar to what would be provided in a skilled nursing facility. Examples of medical services include providing wound care, medicines, or rehabilitation therapy. To be eligible, you must be homebound and only able to leave the house with assistance to go to medical appointments. The agencies providing these services are state regulated, and the service must be ordered by a doctor. They are often Medicare and Medicaid certified. Some non-medical needs, like household chores, dressing, and bathing, can be addressed by an aide, but these services must be done along with medical services being provided. This kind of home health care can be paid for by private health insurance or Medicare, but there is usually the expectation that the need will be temporary as expected improvements take place in the person's medical condition.

The other type of home health is strictly nonmedical in nature and provides help only with household duties and personal care, like meal preparation, bathing, dressing, or moving around the house. Depending on the state, these agencies may or may not be licensed. This type of home health care allows a person with special needs remain at home. It is usually for individuals who are getting older or who are chronically ill or disabled. This type of home care by itself is rarely covered by health insurance. Though this care is paid for without health insurance, it is often less expensive than care provided in a nursing facility setting. Programs that will help with the cost include reverse mortgages, VA benefits, and long-term care insurance. Many states now have waiver programs to afford this care that specifically assist low-income seniors who qualify for Medicaid. These programs provide care at home in order to avoid an admission to a nursing home.

So what is the criteria for evaluating a home care agency?

Longevity – the longer an agency has operated in the community, the longer they have had time to establish a reputation and are thus more likely to be stable. It will therefore be easier to get feedback from past and current clients.

Reputation and Credentials – it is also good to know if the agency is bonded or certified with the state. To check reputation, it is good to get at least one former and one current customer to provide feedback on the service they have received. You should be looking for timeliness of service, respect for the client, and education they provide both about your condition and the role of your caregiver. Another important aspect of reputation is how they are known within the medical community. Because they have to work with your physicians to carry out the treatment plan, it is important to determine whether your physician has successfully worked with that facility in the past.

Staff – who is really providing the care? You want to know the credentials of the people that the agency hires. Does the service hire registered nurses? Are there aides who help with tasks such as bathing or general hygiene? Is there a dietician? What is the hiring process, and how are the personnel screened? Ask what training the agency provides to its caregivers and if the home care aides are certified by the agency. Does the agency require that its caregivers participate in a continuing education program? Ask if the caregivers are trained to identify and report changes in service needs and health condition. Do the caregivers have experience or receive special training in the type of care which is needed, such as Alzheimer's care? Or training with a particular type of assistive technology, such as a Hoyer lift? How long have they been working in the home care field? Does a medical professional or experienced supervisor evaluate and supervise the caregiver in the client's home and get input from the client?

Carrying out the care plan – Does the agency seek input from the client on his/her care plans? Can the agency assure that the same caregiver(s) will provide the home care services each week? How long do caregivers stay with the agency? What is the turnover rate? If a substitute caregiver is going to be sent, when does the agency provide notice to the client? Ask how the agency assures that the substitute caregiver will be familiar with the care plan and individual needs of the client and the family. Does the agency provide a twenty-four emergency phone line? And finally, ask if there are additional costs are not included in the price quoted.

During the interview process, while helping one family find a home care agency for their mother, we found an agency that passed the above screens and also used a personality inventory to match their caregivers with their potential clients. This helped to ensure that the "fit" was right and increased the opportunity for a good bond to be formed. Extras like this may be beneficial in finding the right person to provide assistance.

A Word about Caregiving

Until you go through it, no one really understands the potential demands of providing care for a loved one. But it helps to be as prepared as possible for this very important job in order to help in your loved one's recovery and to be able to continue to tend to your own well-being.

Caregiving is a multilayered and complex job. It can involve some combination of all of the following: providing grooming and hygiene, including bathing, dressing, and toileting; household chores like cooking, shopping for medications/supplies/food, and doing laundry; medical assistance, including everything from wound care to administering medications; and providing companionship, since having an illness is isolating, and the emotional aspect of rehabilitation is just as important as the physical part. Because of these multiple responsibilities, it can be easy for a caregiver to become overwhelmed. It can be difficult to take care of your own self and your obligations while also managing someone else's full time, especially when the situation has occurred with little or no warning.

The best defense, as they say, is a good offense. Early on, during the discharge planning process, or before if possible, determine who among friends and family members will be in charge of providing care after the hospitalization. This not only involves identifying who is the primary-care giver, but also who will be their backup person and how often so they can have a break. These individuals will often have to rearrange work and personal schedules to be able to take care of the steps outlined above and receive caregiving training from hospital personnel. This will provide the opportunity to get used to the more medical parts of care giving – like giving injections, dressing wounds, and operating monitoring devices. It also allows the caregiver(s) to become clear about their loved one's daily needs, learn the particulars of the illness, and develop a relationship with the doctor so they can be a mediator post-discharge. In addition, during this time, assess living quarters to determine if they need to be adjusted for comfort and ease of access. As you go through this caregiver preparation process, it is important to budget in time for your own needs and well-being since staying well yourself is the only way to successfully help others.

Takeaway Checklist

While we may not always be able to plan for a hospital stay, there are steps to take to try to maximize the success of our stay and make our transition out of the hospital a smooth one.

The Hospital Stay

☐ Reference hospital quality websites for the highly ranked hospitals in your area.

☐ Know and communicate your health history and medications with hospital staff caring for you.

☐ Know and communicate the game plan with the hospital staff caring for you. Recognize that it can be adjusted frequently as your condition changes.

☐ Double-check labels – the one on your wrist and on all medications you are given.

☐ Be vocal about your needs.

☐ If you can, prepare your body prior to your hospital stay. This can speed recovery.

☐ Insist on cleanliness and cleansing of hands and instruments like stethoscopes that contact you.

☐ Bring an advocate with you – if possible, someone should be with you as much as is allowed by hospital policy.

Preparing for Discharge

☐ Know how to contact each physician member of your health-care team.

☐ Request an occupational and/or physical therapy consult prior to leaving the hospital if you have had a complex condition or long stay – the result will help you prepare for the next step after the hospital.

☐ Check with your insurance company after your stay to make sure the services you need are covered.

☐ If going home, have a plan for who will help you there and any adjustments needed to your living space.

At Discharge

☐ Get a written list of all tests, procedures, and treatments that were done, their results, and follow-up treatments or procedures that need to be scheduled.

☐ Go over with the doctor or nurse all your medications prior to leaving the hospital – know how they interact with what you were taking prior to entering the hospital.

☐ Make sure there is a follow-up appointment scheduled within seven days with your personal physician and any other physicians involved in the hospital care.

☐ Have a list of the medical supplies you may need if going home and have the corresponding prescriptions. Get a direct telephone number for issues or concerns relating to any equipment.

☐ Know the warning signs of potential problems, including when to call the doctor or go to the ER.

☐ Know the diet you should follow and the specifics of how to care for yourself after leaving the hospital.

☐ Get a list of support groups that specialize in your illness as well as any organizations that provide counseling for the needs of caregivers.

Choosing a Rehabilitation or Skilled Nursing Facility

☐ Get recommendations for a rehabilitation or skilled nursing facility from the hospital case manager or insurance case manager.

☐ Check for quality ratings on Medicare.gov.

☐ Ask the following questions to evaluate the type of care provided:

☐ Why was this type of facility suggested?

☐ What specific medical needs does this facility address?

☐ Can this facility meet all my needs or will additional assistance be necessary?

☐ How close and convenient is this facility for the family and caregiver to visit?

☐ Is it clean, quiet, and comfortable?

☐ Does this facility address any specific nutritional, cultural, or language-related issues?

☐ What is the staff to resident ratio?

☐ Do residents get the assistance they need in a timely fashion?

☐ Does the staff listen attentively and respectfully to residents?

☐ Does the atmosphere appear homelike or is it institutional?

Choosing a Home-Health Agency

☐ Understand prior to hospital discharge whether you will need a skilled home-care agency or one that only addresses non-medical needs.

☐ Evaluate quality through

    o feedback from past and current clients and, if skilled, physicians who have worked with them;

    o requesting the credentials of staff, screening procedures for hiring, and the training and supervision they get;

    o understanding how the care is provided – is there continuity of care with the caregiver provided, is the care plan tailored to each client's individual needs, and how do new caregivers learn the care plan.

    o knowing whether the agency provides a twenty-four emergency phone line?

☐ Are additional costs not included in the price quoted?

Caregiving

☐ Determine who among friends and family members will be in charge of providing care after the hospitalization . . . and their back-up person.

☐ Ensure that the caregiver gets educated about how care needs to be provided at home prior to leaving the hospital.

☐ Ensure the caregiver budgets in time for their own needs and well-being.

Should You Consider a Clinical Trial?

*If we knew what it was we were doing, it
would not be called research, would it?*

– Albert Einstein

Just this year, there was a news report of Rabbi Refoel Shmulevitz being the first known individual with a reversal of the symptoms of amyotrophic lateral sclerosis (ALS), otherwise known as Lou Gehrig's disease. What did he do differently? Diagnosed with ALS two years ago, he was confined to a wheelchair, with limited ability to speak and breathe, and suffering with another rare disease, Myasthenia Gravis. He was treated with an experimental stem cell therapy that is still in clinical trials. Per the report, within a few weeks following injection with the stem cells, his breathing, speech, walking, muscular strength, and overall well-being improved.

E VERY ONCE IN a while, we hear about new treatments like this that potentially offer hope for hard-to-treat diseases. These treatments are first tested through a process called clinical trials before they can be approved for use in the general population. So why do people consider participating in clinical trials? And what are they all about anyway?

What Is a Clinical Trial?

Clinical trials are research studies done with human volunteers that are designed to answer specific health questions and to find treatments that work. Researchers test whether new drugs or devices are safe for use in people, whether the treatment can be tolerated, and, finally, if it works well. But not only new treatments are tested. Sometimes existing standard treatments are compared to each other to determine which one is better; or improvements to standard treatments are tested to see if they can be made more effective, easier to use, or have fewer side effects. Finally, studies can be done to learn how to best use a standard treatment in a new population, such as children, where it has not been used before.

The Food and Drug Administration (FDA) sets the rules to make sure that people who agree to be in studies are treated as safely as possible. Following severe ethical violations that ended only forty years ago in the infamous Tuskegee Syphilis Experiments, the federal government established regulations and guidelines for clinical research to protect participants. Researchers have to adhere to these federal regulations in order to conduct research. One strict requirement is to explain to potential participants, through a process called informed consent, the potential risks and benefits or participation in the trial. Researchers must also review your rights as a research participant, which include the ability to withdraw from participating in the trial at any time.

The Tuskegee Syphilis Experiments was an infamous research study conducted between 1932 and 1972 by the U.S. Public Health Service to study the natural progression of untreated *syphilis* in rural black men. The men were led to believe they were receiving free health care from the U.S. government but never received treatment for their disease.

How to Evaluate If a Clinical Trial Is for You

So are clinical trials for you? They are an option that can be considered if standard treatments just are not working for you, either because of unacceptable side effects or just a lack of improvement. You may also have a health condition for which there is no effective cure, like ALS or dementia. Some people participate in trials solely because they want to contribute to the advancement of medical knowledge.

Potential benefits to being in a well-designed and well-executed clinical trial include gaining access to potentially new research treatments, having access to experts in the field for your condition, and contributing to medical research. Possible risks include unpleasant, serious, or even life-threatening side effects resulting from the treatment; a lack of positive effect for the participant; additional time and effort beyond what the standard treatment involves, like visits to the study site on a regular basis, getting more treatments, evaluations, and tests that are normally necessary or staying in the hospital for additional time.

If you decide that you want to identify any clinical trials out there that you could participate in, how do you go about finding them? There is more than one way to go about it. The possibilities include:

1. ClinicalTrials.gov – You can find information about current clinical trials by searching this interactive online database managed by the National Library of Medicine. It provides information about both federally and privately supported clinical research in human volunteers. ClinicalTrials.gov is updated regularly and offers information on each trial's

purpose, eligibility rules for participation, locations for enrollment, and phone numbers to call for more information.

2. Your health-care professional – Sometimes your doctor, especially if he or she is a specialist, gets information about clinical trials being conducted. Even if they do not know about one, you can ask them to help you find one for which you would qualify.

3. Condition specific organizations/foundations – Nonprofit organizations devoted to finding treatments and resources for single conditions, like the Lupus Foundation of America or the America Diabetes Association, often have information about ongoing clinical trials for their respective conditions.

When you do find a clinical trial that may be of interest to you, there are some key things you should get answers about before considering joining one. These answers are usually available from talking with the study coordinator and in the informed consent document.

1. **What is the protocol?** Clinical trials are conducted according to a plan called a protocol. The protocol describes what types of patients may enter the study, schedules of tests and procedures, drugs, dosages, and length of study as well as the outcomes that will be measured. You should have a detailed understanding of exactly what will happen during the study. Each person participating in the study must agree to the rules set out by the protocol. It is also important to know that not everyone who applies for a clinical trial will meet the criteria for participation.

2. **Does everyone get the treatment being tested?** Many clinical trials are designed so that one group of people gets the treatment being tested, and another, the comparison or control group does not get the treatment. The comparison group not receiving the treatment gets a placebo, an inactive substitute for the treatment, so that the differences in outcomes between the two groups can be compared. When you enroll in these kinds of trials, you are randomly assigned to a group, so there is no way to know ahead of time what group you will be in. Depending on the trial design, you could have anywhere from a 90-10 chance of being in the treatment group to a 50-50 chance. The researchers in charge of the trial should explain what your chances are based on the study design.

3. **What are the risks of that particular protocol?** Some risks may be unavoidable because of the uncertainty inherent in medical research studies involving new treatments. Risks include any pain or discomfort as well as potential side effects. The government requires researchers to give prospective participants complete and accurate information about what will happen during the trial. Participants must sign an informed consent document before joining the study, indicating they understand that the trial is research and that they can leave the clinical trial at any time. This informed consent document details the exact known risks associated with the study and any potential unknown risks of the product being studied. This information is essential for you to know if you want to enroll in the clinical trial based on the level of risk involved.

4. **What is the potential time frame during which side effects can surface?** Sometimes the study protocol may only look at potential effects for a short period of time. However, if there can be longer-term effects, you should know what they are and the time frame in which may become apparent.

5. **Who is the sponsor?** Clinical trials can be sponsored by an organization such as a pharmaceutical company, a federal agency like the National Institutes of Health or Veterans Administration, or an individual, such as a physician or health-care provider. The sponsor determines the locations of the trial which can be universities, medical centers, clinics, doctor's offices, hospitals, and/or federally and industry funded research sites.

6. **Do you stay on your regular medications while in the study?** If you do not stay on your regular medications, you should discuss any potential concerns about stopping them with your regular doctor. If you continue your regular medicines, you should know if there any anticipated negative interactions between what you are getting on the study protocol, including any anesthesia, and what you are already taking.

7. **What financial costs are there related to participation, and will the study cover any of them?** You should understand any potential costs you might have to pay. These can include the cost of the product, costs associated with administering the product, lab or X-ray testing, and travel and lodging costs associated with getting to the study site. Some of these costs may be covered by the study

itself. In addition, individuals are sometimes paid for their participation in research, especially in the early phases of investigational drugs or devices. Financial incentives are sometimes used when health benefits to subjects are remote or nonexistent, when there is considerable time required, and/or for any discomfort that may be experienced during the trial. Payment information, including the amount and schedule of payment(s) as well as any possible costs to volunteers who participate in a study are discussed with potential participants during the informed consent process and documented in the informed consent form.

8. **Will your insurance pay for any of the costs of the trial?** Some insurance companies will pay for any testing or treatment connected with a clinical trial that is considered standard care. This generally means that they might cover everything short of the cost of the experimental drug and costs of administering it. Remember that any costs you bear associated with your treatment are tax deductible if they are beyond a certain percentage of your annual income. So save any and all study-related receipts, including medical costs, travel, lodging, and food.

9. **Does your health-care professional get paid a fee for recommending, referring, or enrolling patients in the trial?** You should know if your health-care provider will receive monetary compensation for referring you to a clinical trial. This is a legitimate way the clinical studies use to find participants. However, it is important if you want an unbiased opinion as to whether you should participate. If your provider is receiving compensation for referring you,

you should get advice elsewhere about whether to enroll in the trial.

10. **Will the treatment be stopped at the end of the trial even if it was proven beneficial?** Some sponsors continue to provide product. Others do not. You should find this out and understand how you will be able to have continuing access to the treatment.

Takeaway Checklist

☐ Discuss with your doctor if a clinical trial may be right for you. If you doctor gets incentives for referrals, get a second opinion from a specialist physician not involved in the trial

☐ To find a clinical trial, check www.clinicaltrials.gov, ask your doctor, or ask a representative from a foundation or association that focuses on the condition you have.

☐ If considering a specific clinical trial, talk with the study coordinator or lead investigator about the following:

    ☐ What is the protocol?

    ☐ Does everyone get the treatment being tested?

    ☐ What are the risks of that particular protocol?

    ☐ What is the potential time frame during which side effects can surface?

    ☐ Who is the sponsor?

    ☐ Do you stay on your regular medications while in the study?

    ☐ What financial costs are there related to participation and will the study cover any of them?

☐ Will your insurance pay for any of the costs of the trial?

☐ Does your health-care professional get paid a fee for recommending, referring, or enrolling patients in the trial?

☐ Will the treatment be stopped at the end of the trial even if proved to be beneficial?

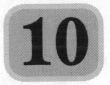

Financing Your Care

A hospital bed is a parked taxi with the meter running.

– Groucho Marx

I consulted with young man who had been stabbed in a fight when he tried to help a friend who was being jumped. Luckily, the stab wound seemed to be superficial after a wound exploration done in the emergency trauma unit. The trauma surgeon recommended keeping him in the hospital overnight to observe him to make sure that he had no bowel injury that would later reveal itself. He felt fine and wanted to go home, but his mom persuaded him to stay. The hospital bill for his overnight stay, emergency visit, and consultation was over $5,000. Being only twenty-two years old, he did not have this kind of money and chose to ignore the bill. Ignoring the bill led to it going to collections and ruining his credit. Six years later, he is still feeling the effects of poor credit which has led to his inability to get a home loan for his now young family, and he has never been able to have a credit card with an interest rate lower than 18 percent, further compounding his problems.

ONE OF THE greatest difficulties with our present health-care system is the cost. Over 1.5 million people will experience financial crises due to medical expenses, just like the young man with whom I consulted. And he is one of the relative lucky ones since he never had to declare bankruptcy or foreclosure. In the U.S., debt due to medical bills is the leading cause of home foreclosures. But given the high cost of health care, it is no wonder that over half of all foreclosures are caused by medical hardship. Health-care costs for a family of four topped $20,000 in 2012. Those with employers paid about $8,500 of that ($3,500 out of pocket and

$5,000 in payroll deductions for premiums) while the employer picked up the remainder. The total monthly cost works out to about the average family's monthly mortgage payment of $1,670. And the increase in health-care costs is triple that of inflation, so we have not seen the upper limit of how high costs will continue to rise. In addition to foreclosure and debt, the consequence of these runaway costs is people skipping or delaying getting the care they need.

This chapter covers what you need to know about affording and getting good health care. It covers paying for both complementary and conventional services, whether you are insured, trying to buy insurance, or uninsured; how to manage your health insurance company, get the most from the services they offer, and what to do if they do not come through; and finally, what resources are available to help you pay for services you need but may not be able to afford, like medications, lab tests, professional fees, hospital bills, copays, and deductibles.

Health Insurance – Getting It and Making It Work for You

Health insurance is protection against medical expenses you would not be able to easily afford on your own. Almost 85 percent of Americans have some kind of health insurance. About 31 percent of individuals are covered by public sources, mostly Medicare and Medicaid, while employers cover just over 55 percent of individuals. Just over 15 percent of Americans – nearly 50 million individuals – were uninsured in 2010. If you are now in a position to get health insurance – either buying coverage yourself or selecting a plan at work – what should you know about selecting a plan? Once you have health insurance, do you know how to minimize costs while getting the services you need? And if you run into problems with your insurance plan refusing to cover needed services, what do you do?

How Do I Figure Out What Type of Insurance I Need?

Let us start with getting the right plan for you. Whether you are getting insurance through your job or individually, there are some basic principles to keep in mind. They all revolve around knowing and anticipating the health needs of you and your family for the upcoming year. If you or someone in your family has been diagnosed with a chronic condition, you will likely have doctor visits, possible ER and hospital visits, lab work, X-rays, and medications. You may want the flexibility to go to the best hospitals and doctors you can find, and you may want to seek out alternative and complementary care too. Additionally, other family members may only need preventive and screening services. You want to choose a plan that allows for all these different health-care transactions while minimizing the amount you will pay out of pocket. So let's see what we need to look for. Before we get into the checklist of what you should consider when choosing an insurance plan, let's talk about how most health insurance plans are structured.

Indemnity Plans

Indemnity plans, also called fee-for-service or reimbursement plans, allow you to see any doctor you want anytime you want. You pay the doctor directly and then send your claim to your insurance company. The company pays you back for part of the total cost. (For example, if your doctor charged $100, you might get 75 percent or $75 back.) Because they offer you the most choice, the monthly premium is usually higher than other types of health plans. In the past, indemnity plans did not pay for preventive care, which included basic items like annual physical exams, screening tests, and vaccines. However, because of health-care reform, starting in 2010, insurance companies now have to cover most preventive services. Health-care reform also has changed the annual limit on total costs for the year. Previously, plans would not cover charges above a certain preset spending limit. As a result of health-care reform, most plans have had to remove these limits.

Managed Care Plans

When you get insurance through an employer, it is often through a managed care plan, similar to Kaiser Permanente. However, these same managed care plans are also available for individuals on the open market. With managed care, a health insurance company negotiates a contract with certain health-care providers, hospitals, and labs to provide care for its members at a lower cost. There are three major types of managed care plans.

1. **HMO (Health Maintenance Organization).** When you join an HMO, you choose a primary-care doctor – an internist, family medicine doctor, or a pediatrician. This doctor coordinates all your medical care, from annual physicals to hospitalizations. The great thing about HMOs is they tend to be the lowest for premiums and out-of-pocket expenses. Doctor's visits, preventive care, and medical

treatment are covered by your monthly insurance premium, and there is no individual or family deductible to meet. There is generally a copayment for each visit that varies based on the type of service provided and the plan you select but typically no coinsurance. However, what you give up is flexibility, because you can only use doctors and hospitals who are approved by your plan. Also, you cannot see a specialist without a written referral from your primary-care doctor. This is not true for emergency-room visits, since by law, emergency care cannot be restricted; however, emergency care usually requires a higher copay.

2. **PPO (Preferred Provider Organization).** A PPO offers greater flexibility than an HMO. Instead of having a designated primary-care doctor who controls your access to specialists, you can see any doctor you want. By choosing a doctor who participates in your plan, you will have a lower copayment than if you see a doctor outside of the plan. If you do choose to stray from your PPO network, you may need to pay for the treatment and submit the receipt to your PPO insurance provider for a partial reimbursement. Finally, some PPO plans have coinsurance, not to be confused with a copayment. A copayment or copay is typically a fixed cost based on the type of visit, the type of provider, and whether the provider is in or out of network. Coinsurance is designed for you, the insured, to share the cost with the insurer. It is a percentage of the insurance that you pay after the deductible is met until you reach the policy's designated out-of-pocket limit. For example, Keenan had a 20 percent coinsurance clause on his health insurance policy. The total bill for his hospitalization for a heart attack was $20,000. His health

insurance deductible was $2,000 for the year. This means that Keenan pays out of his pocket the deductible ($2,000), and then 20 percent of the remaining amount of the insurance bill which is $3,600 ($20,000–$2,000=$18,000 x 20%). So the total out-of-pocket expense is $5,600 ($2,000+$3,600). The policy out-of-pocket limit for Keenan is $5,600, so any covered health-care cost for the rest of the year is paid for 100 percent by the health plan.

3. **POS (Point of Service).** A POS plan is just like a HMO-PPO hybrid. You are generally required to choose a primary care in-network doctor for most of your care, just like an HMO, but you may go outside the network if you need to see a specialist, like the PPO. If you do go out of network, you have to pay more.

Consumer-Driven Health Plan (CDHP)

Consumer-driven health plans, also called high-deductible health plans, are fairly new and were developed so that employers could shift more of the costs onto employees. The downside of course is a much-higher contribution. The benefit is that is gives the employee more discretion over how to spend their money. They all generally work like this: (1) an employer pays a fixed amount toward each employee's health benefits; (2) each employee has an untaxed health account that they control and use to pay health-care bills – including costs that a traditional health plan might not cover, like alternative medicine visits. These are usually called Health Savings Accounts or HSAs; (3) unspent money in the account rolls over from year to year if not spent; (4) the deductibles and copays are high, and the health insurance basically ends up paying for major expenses;

and (5) the employee gets online support to track health-care bills, maintain health, get information on provider quality, and get discounted prices. This type of plan may work if you are basically healthy, just need preventive services, which are mostly covered, and may want to use your money for things your health insurance would not have paid for anyway – cosmetic procedures, alternative care, and over-the-counter medicines. If you have an illness, though, you will have to go through your entire deductible and considerable amount of coinsurance before your plan kicks in to help.

There are two main variations of the accounts associated with consumer-driven health plans – the Health Reimbursement Account (HRA) and the Health Savings Account (HSA).

- **Health Reimbursement Accounts (HRAs).** Only employers can set up an HRA, the company makes all the contributions, and the employer owns the account. The company can reclaim any unspent balance, though most employers let the money roll over from year to year.
- **Health Savings Accounts (HSAs).** An individual or employer can setup an HSA and both can contribute tax-free dollars to it. The key is that you, as the employee, own the money even if it was set up by the employer and includes employer contributions. Money rolls over from year to year, and the interest income in the account remains untaxed. There are yearly caps on how much you can contribute which increase slightly if you are age fifty-five to sixty-five.

Note – while these are similar to medical Flexible Spending Accounts (FSA), the HSA and HRA are only associated with consumer-driven health plans. FSAs can be offered by an employer with traditional health insurance plans. FSAs let you set aside money tax free from your paycheck to pay for uncovered but approved medical expenses such as deductibles, copayments, dental and vision care, and some alternative treatments. You can even take an advance against funds you plan to set aside by the end of the year. For example, you can pay for a qualified medical expense of $1,000 with only $400 in your FSA by borrowing against future deposits. On the downside, if you lose or quit your job, you lose any unspent FSA funds. In addition, you must track your medical expenses carefully and submit proof to justify payments. Your employee benefit office can provide a clear explanation of which expenses are eligible under your FSA and which are not. The Affordable Care Act has changed limited FSAs in two ways. You can no longer use money in your FSA to pay for over-the-counter drugs unless you get a doctor's prescription first. And the maximum amount you can set aside will be capped at $2,500 in 2013, which was previously determined by your employer to be up to $5,000.

So what are the three key items you need to ask yourself when looking at an insurance plan?

1. **What will I have to pay?** Consider all aspects of the plan when figuring this out, not just the monthly cost of the plan or the premium. You also must factor in the deductible – the amount you pay out of pocket before the insurance kicks in; the copay, your portion of the bill, which is usually a flat fee, like $35 for every emergency department visits or $10 of the cost of every office visit; and the coinsurance percentage, if there is one. Lastly, consider too if the plan comes with an HRA, FSA, or HSA since this will affect your taxable income and cover some expenses. Make sure

the premium is one you can afford each month. However, know that, generally, the higher your premium, the lower your deductible. For example, a plan with a low monthly premium is not necessarily the cheapest – your copay might be very high, or you might have to go through a $5,000 deductible before your insurance actually kicks in. If you see a doctor a lot or take prescription medications regularly, a more expensive plan that covers a higher percentage of the cost for services or medicines may actually turn out to be cheaper. Also important to know is if there is a limit on your coinsurance or copay for the year. This is important so that you will not go bankrupt paying for your portion of the bill if there is no copay limit or if the limit is way beyond what you can afford. Fortunately, there are some organizations, which we will cover later, that help with copays and coinsurance for those who cannot afford it. It is best not to attempt to lower your premium by selecting a plan that omits major benefit categories, such as prescription drugs. Instead, you can lower your premium with a higher deductible (like $2,500 rather than $1,000), a higher out-of-pocket limit (say $10,000 rather than $7,500), or both. So when you are healthy, you might get little or no benefit from your policy. But the policy will do what it is designed for which is to provide protection against financial ruin due to high medical bills. For people buying any type of health insurance on their own, the website *ehealthinsurance.com* estimates that savings are more for older individuals than younger ones. For example, a twenty-five-year-old man can expect to save only about $900 on the premium by switching from a $500 deductible to a $5,000 deductible, a savings of $912. But for a fifty-five-year-old man, making the same change would yield a savings of $2,040.

Table 1: What You Have To Pay Questions:
What is the premium?
What is the deductible?
Is there a copay or coinsurance?
Is there a limit to what I will have to pay, and can I afford up to that limit if needed?

---

2. **What does the plan cover?** A comprehensive policy is one that covers doctors' visits, outpatient treatments like chemotherapy, diagnostic and screening tests and procedures, prescription drugs, hospital care, emergency services, mental health services, substance abuse treatment, laboratory and imaging tests, preventive care, maternity care, and rehabilitation services. Depending on your needs, you should also check to see if your plan covers additional services – like counseling, chiropractic, acupuncture, vision or dental – that may be important to you. Plans that cover these may have higher premiums, but if you expect to use these services, the extra cost might be worth it to you. If alternative medicine is very important, your state insurance department may be able to help you determine which insurance companies cover complementary medicine. In addition, professional associations for alternative medicine specialties may monitor insurance coverage and reimbursement in their field. You can consult them via their websites for advice.

3. **Does this plan provide the flexibility I want?** You pay for flexibility. Flexibility means the option to choose what doctors you want to see without having to get a referral from a primary-care doctor. You and your family may be mostly healthy and decide that based on what you can afford, a high degree of choice in doctors and hospitals is not a priority. If you are accessing mainly preventive services, then the restrictions of going to a designated primary physician for referrals and staying in a network are not an issue. An HMO might be for you. If you have an ongoing illness or new symptoms that need evaluation, choice becomes more important. The savings of going with a high-deductible health plan that gives lots of choice compared with a standard HMO or PPO plan can vary substantially depending on your age and medical circumstances and what area of the country you live in. For example, in a national survey of job-based health insurance plans, the worker's share of the annual family coverage premium for a high-deductible HSA plan was $3,457 compared with $4,357 for an HMO – a savings of $900. But if the high-deductible HSA plan had a deductible of $5,000 and the HMO deductible was only $1,000, that saving is rapidly eaten up once you start to access services.

Buying Individual Coverage and the 2014 Health Insurance Marketplace

The entire search for individual health insurance for those with preexisting conditions will soon be different, thanks to the

Affordable Care Act (ACA). When key parts of the ACA take effect in 2014, there will be a new way to get health insurance: the Health Insurance Marketplace. Any U.S. national or citizen living in the U.S. is eligible to use the new marketplace. Every health insurance plan in the new marketplace is prescreened and will offer comprehensive coverage. It will be simple to compare various insurance options based on price, benefits, and quality. Under the health-care law, there will also be new protections. Health insurance companies will no longer be able to refuse to cover you or charge more just because you have a chronic or preexisting condition. They also cannot charge more to insure women versus men. Open enrollment starts October 2013. Coverage starts January 1, 2014. Visit **www.healthcare.gov** to learn more about the marketplace.

However, until then, individuals buying health coverage on their own have to be especially careful about avoiding inadequate health plans. Individually purchased plans are also more expensive because no employer is involved who can offset the cost. Plans that seem to promise too much, offer big discounts with low premiums, link their product to the new health-care reform law or guarantee acceptance, especially if your health is poor, are all suspect. As a matter of fact, until the health-care reform laws start in 2014, plans can still turn you down or charge more for an individual policy if you have a known illness, also called a preexisting condition. Examples of plans which may not deliver all that they seem to promise include the following:

a. **Limited benefit coverage plans or "minimeds"** – these plans are cheaper because they do not offer the comprehensive coverage that protects you from major expenses. "Undercoverage" may leave you holding the bag when you most need the help. For example, a minimed plan may only pay $800 a day for a hospitalization that actually costs $3,000 or may not cover rehabilitation expenses after a major illness.

b. **No-deductible or extremely low premium plans** – the vast majority of legitimate insurance plans have deductibles, or if they have low premiums, they have high deductibles. Often, plans that advertise no deductible have a low maximum payout and the consumer is left without coverage when they may need it most.

c. **Medical-discount plans** – these plans are not really legitimate insurance. They charge you a monthly fee for a card that supposedly entitles you to discounts from various medical providers. Many of these offer no legitimate discounts, but even the ones that do, neglect to cover medical bills. These discount plans, plus any of the above plans, may include the phrase "not major medical," which is a tip-off that they do not include comprehensive coverage.

d. **Health-care sharing ministries** – these are faith-based organizations that collect monthly shares from participating members that are then distributed to those with medical needs. They have been on the rise as more people have been unable to afford coverage, and faith-based organizations have tried to fill the gap. However, participants in these ministries should understand that it is not insurance because it does not pay providers directly, and there is no binding contract to cover members' expenses. There are also no legal protections available such as with state-regulated insurance products.

So until 2014, where can you go to find a reliable plan? HealthCare.gov is the federal government's insurance information portal. It rates over 11,500 health insurance plans and provides information on costs based on age and gender, the providers in the network, and medications included, also called the drug formulary. You can also see statistics about the number of patients refused coverage or charged extra because of preexisting conditions.

Other options include using an insurance broker who represents multiple plans. Especially if you have a preexisting condition, it helps to apply to multiple plans, and a broker can facilitate this process. Brokers can also request a prescreen from each potential insurer, an anonymous assessment of whether they might insure you and at what cost, based on your health history. Also, state insurance departments can direct you to either state high-risk pools or private insurers mandated by states to provide coverage, regardless of preexisting conditions. This coverage is usually the most expensive.

Finally, the Better Business Bureau and your State Department of Insurance/Insurance Commissioner are reliable sources to check if an insurance plan has had any consumer complaints. The lack of complaints does not guarantee that the insurance plan is without fault; however, multiple complaints are a good indication that you should redirect your efforts to an organization with a better consumer track record.

How to Get the Most Out of
Your Health Insurance Company

There are a few key ways that you can take advantage of your health insurance company offerings once you have purchased insurance individually or through your employer. Many people do not know about these opportunities because they are not well publicized. These opportunities are based upon the fact that insurance companies know that healthy individuals cost less to insure over time. From an insurance company perspective, low-cost members do not use the hospital or the emergency department. They also get scheduled screenings that catch illness early, use treatments and medications as prescribed, and pay attention to staying well.

Consequently, many insurance companies have created programs with incentives to encourage their members to adopt healthy behaviors. Not all insurances have these programs. However, if your health plan does, you may benefit from participation. Participating in these programs requires that you interact with an insurance company nurse or that you enter health information online to your insurance company. Some people are concerned because they feel they are giving their private information to their insurance company which may affect their policy or employability in the future. While you are giving some details, it is important to realize that health insurance companies already have access to all your health information. They get this information every time they pay one of your health-care bills, called claims. Each claim contains tons of information about you – your diagnoses, lab, and X-ray results, medications and how often they have been filled, and every doctor visit, hospitalization, or ER visit you have had. So your insurance company already has a quite comprehensive picture of you. The point of participation in the programs is to keep you healthy and therefore save money for the insurance company or your employer. However, there is clear benefit for you – staying healthy, the potential for less out-of-pocket health-care costs, and additional money in your pocket through the incentives paid. So let's see how this works.

1. **Health Risk Assessments (HRA)** – sometimes your employer or your insurance company will offer you an incentive – like a gift card, a discount on your premium, money in your health savings account, or points that can be redeemed – to fill out what is called a health risk assessment (HRA). An HRA provides an evaluation of risks to your health and quality of life. Typically, there is an extended questionnaire that asks you demographic information like age and gender; lifestyle (exercise, smoking, alcohol intake, diet); personal medical history; physiologic data (weight, height, blood pressure, cholesterol); and attitudes toward health and willingness to change in order to improve health. Some HRAs have questions about family medical history; however, in the U.S., due to the *Genetic Information Nondiscrimination Act* (see table 2), questions regarding family medical history are not permitted if there is any incentive attached to taking an HRA.

Table 2: GINA is a 2008 U.S. Act of Congress that protects individuals from health insurers or employers using their genetic information to deny them insurance coverage or employment, including *hiring, firing,* job placement, or *promotion* decisions.

Genetic Nondiscrimination Federal Legislation Archive. *http://www.genome.gov/11510239 accessed July 28,* 2012

Once this information is entered, a health rating score is calculated that reflects risks to your health. Based on this score, there is some form of feedback provided, often broken down into specific subscores and areas such as stress, nutrition, and fitness. Users get results delivered either in an automatic online report or a discussion with a health advisor. The goal is to provide individualized feedback with at least one intervention to promote health and prevent disease. Most often, HRAs will be Internet-based, either on your employer's or health plan's secure website. You get the incentive once you have filled out the questionnaire. In some cases, depending on your employer's policies, just filing out the HRA and doing nothing else can mean money in your pocket. However, research has shown that following the advice from the HRA can positively impact your health. These incentives are available to members regardless of their health status.

2. **Health coaching** – imagine having your very own coach to help you achieve your health goals – to lose weight, reduce your back pain, get your blood sugar under control, support you through your cancer treatments? What if you could have this for free, provided as a service by your insurance company? Well, many insurances companies do provide coaches for their clients. These health coaches, who generally are licensed nurses, nutritionists, or other health-care professionals are specially trained and certified to help you set your health-related goals, identify barriers, and to support you in changing your lifestyle and choices. And get this! Some even offer you incentives – monetary and otherwise – to participate in the program. Generally, the insurance company will contact you if you have a chronic health condition; however, you or your doctor can refer you into the appropriate program. Most companies only focus

on certain health conditions, like high blood pressure or diabetes, so check to see if your insurance company has a program that fits your health concerns.

3. **Case management/care coordination** – when you suffer a catastrophic illness, where do you turn for help in determining the appropriate services and providers you need to help to you through? The last place you may think of is your insurance company. However, you may be surprised to learn that there are nurses employed by insurance companies who help members get the appropriate services and resources in a cost-effective way. Their concern is quality of care for the member as well as cost. Remember, it is not in the insurance companies' best financial interest for you to just use the cheapest services. They also need for you to get the best quality services within the benefits that you have purchased that will help you regain as much of your health as possible. To that end, the case manager directs you to doctors and services within your benefits and helps you find resources specific to your circumstances throughout in the entire process of getting treatment. While there are rarely incentives for working with a case manager, there can be great benefit in having assistance with coordinating your health-care needs when you have been disabled by illness.

4. **Health Navigation Services**: These services are similar to case management in that they are provided by nurses but are available even if you do not have a life-changing illness. You may just need to know what questions to ask your doctor before going in for surgery or where to go to get the right diagnosis for puzzling symptoms. A health navigation program can help answer your health-care-related questions

and plan a health budget with or without a catastrophic illness. In addition to chatting with nurses, online apps are available to help with health-care decision making, such as getting elective surgery.

How to Avoid and Deal with Denial of Coverage

When you are seeking to have a specialized medical service, insurance companies review these requests to decide if they will cover the costs involved, a process called precertification or preauthorization. Common services reviewed include procedures, hospitalization, costly medications or medical equipment, and rehabilitation services. Let's review the common scenarios and reasons why an insurance company will deny payment. Then we will see what you can do to either avoid getting into these situations or effectively address them if they come up.

1. **A Mistake:** Mistakes happen. Behind all the decisions made at your insurance company are individuals who sometimes make mistakes. Because of this, I encourage you to question any denied payment. Recently, when my husband had an overnight stay in the hospital, payment was denied for the doctor who saw him the next morning before he was discharged. Upon questioning this decision, the insurance company representative said it was because the bill was for an outpatient visit to an out-of-network doctor. When I explained that this doctor saw my husband while he was hospitalized and not as an outpatient, they apologized, resubmitted the bill, and it was paid.

2. **Benefit Not Covered:** A common reason for denial of payment is that the insurance company does not cover a particular service. Every insurance company issues its members a document that lists what is and is not covered. This document generally has a name, like Evidence of Coverage, Plan Description, or Benefit Summary, and is basically your contract with them. There generally is a section that describes the types of services that are *not* covered – for example, it may be called "Exclusions". If a treatment or service, like fertility treatments or liposuction, is listed as not covered, you can pretty much count on it not being covered. It is *extremely* rare to never that an insurance company will make any exceptions unless the situation is extreme such as an immediate life-threatening condition. Common conditions not covered include some alternative health services like reiki; procedures solely to improve appearance, called cosmetic procedures, such as liposuction or hair removal; and services for convenience that do not meet a medical need, like care in the home if you are not homebound.

3. **Not Meeting "Medical Necessity Criteria":** If the service or treatment you are seeking is one that can be covered, your particular case still must meet the insurance company criteria of being "medically necessary." Medical necessity means that without the treatment, your health would suffer. Insurance companies use a set of very specific predetermined criteria to decide whether a particular service or treatment qualifies as being medically needed. Providers generally submit a request on your behalf that includes your medical information relevant to the procedure. It can take up to three weeks to

get a decision back unless it is for an urgent intervention, which can be decided within forty-eight hours or even the same day. It is best not to schedule a procedure until you have confirmed that it will be covered. There are several scenarios where this process can end up resulting in a denial for your request:

a. Medical Criteria: You do not meet the medical criteria for the treatment being provided – for example, your doctor wants to treat you with Botox for your migraines, but the insurance criteria requires that you have tried other medicines first (usually ones that are less expensive) before they will agree to pay for Botox.

b. Investigational or experimental therapies: The insurance does not cover the requested medical treatment or procedure because it has not been proven through research to be effective. For example, you may be getting a treatment that is experimental or not standard, such as stem cell therapy for Alzheimer's disease. Generally, insurance companies require published studies that have evaluated a significant number of people on the treatment over several months to years, showing it is effective and safe. Only these treatments are considered standard and will be reimbursed.

c. Specific situations

1. Hospital Stays – if you are admitted to a hospital, the days you stay there may not be paid for by your insurance. This could be because of medical criteria reasons – doctors and nurses must clearly

record how sick you are and the care you are getting every day, such as IV medicines or fluids, advanced monitoring, and complex wound care. If these treatments are not clearly recorded, your stay may be denied. A denial may also occur if the care you are getting is not the standard care provided by most doctors for your condition – it is experimental, for example. Finally, all or part of the stay can be denied because the hospital is not providing you services in a timely fashion. For example, your hospital stay is prolonged because there were no operating rooms available for two days, or the specialist did not come in over the weekend to perform the special procedure you needed. Most often, denials of hospital admissions or days in the hospital are due to reasons out of your control. The crazy thing is, in these instances, the hospital will bill you for the days that the insurance company did not pay for, even though it may have been due to the doctors' or the hospitals' failure to act. We will see later how to address these.

2. Stays in a Rehabilitation Facility – insurance companies expect that the care you receive while in rehab facility (also called a skilled nursing facility or nursing home) will result in your condition improving. If not improving, you must at least be getting advanced nursing care, like complex wound care or frequent IV medicines, which are not simple enough to administer at

home. You risk having your stay not reimbursed in the following scenarios – you are not improving, you have no complex nursing needs, or your rehab can occur safely at home (you are not bed bound, and your balance is good enough so you will not fall and hurt yourself). However, the most common scenario for your stay in a skilled facility being denied is that your insurance company limits the number of days it will reimburse for rehabilitation. Depending on the insurance policy, it is usually thirty to forty-five days. It is important to check your policy early in the stay to know the limit.

So how do you avoid these scenarios of coverage or medical necessity denials that could be financially disastrous? They also occur at the worse time – when you are trying to recover from an illness and really do not need the extra stress of worrying about money. Let's go over some prevention techniques as well as ways to address the situation if, heaven forbid, it does happen to you.

General Principles of Making Sure You Get Your Insurance Needs Met

1. Know your Plan Description document well so that you will know what the insurance benefits are and what is not covered. If your doctor proposes a particular treatment, piece of equipment, or medication, look it up before agreeing to it. Otherwise, you may get stuck with the bill if it is not covered.

2. Communicate all relevant information to your doctor before he or she submits your request for a particular service. Here are some common scenarios and the information your doctor needs to know and include in your request:

    o   If you want an elective procedure (such as a hysterectomy, weight loss surgery, or back surgery) – your doctor and you should have tried all standard options short of surgery. Depending on your condition, standard options can include medication, physical therapy, weight loss, exercise, counseling, consultations with specialty physicians, braces just to name a few. The doctor should document how the condition you are trying to remedy has caused significant problems in your life.

    o   For genetic tests (such as those to identify cancer patterns in families) – provide as many details about your family's health history as possible

    o   If you are seeking a treatment for pain – make sure you let your doctor know how long you have had the pain, what you have tried to relieve it, and how it affects your ability to carry out your daily activities

    o   If you are requesting a new medicine – make sure that you and your doctor have first tried all the standard medicines recognized to treat your condition, especially if the medicine you are requesting now is new on the market for your condition. If there are reasons why you in particular cannot take a certain medicine, this should be clearly recorded. For example, the standard treatment for heartburn is Carafate, but if you are allergic to it or

have unsuccessfully tried it, you may need one of the
more expensive medications.

o   Experimental and investigational – make sure that
you ask your doctor if the treatment he plans to use,
especially if it is new, is one that is approved by the
FDA for its stated purpose and has some established
track record. Otherwise, you have risk getting it turned
down for reimbursement by your insurance company.

3.   Ensure your doctor submits the request for a medication,
piece of equipment, or service to your insurance company as
soon as it is clear that you need it. The approval process can
take up to three weeks in some instances.

4.   Ensure your doctor is familiar with your insurance company's
detailed guidelines for determining medical necessity. If he is
not, these guidelines are available upon request. Most large
insurance companies, such as United, Cigna, Humana, and
Aetna Inc., post their medical policies online. By reviewing
the guidelines ahead of time, you and your provider can
know immediately if you meet the requirements and, if not,
see what you need to do to meet them.

5.   Know if preauthorization is required based on the item or on
the cost. If your request is for a piece of equipment, like a
sleep apnea machine or wheelchair, find out whether your
insurance company requires prior authorization specifically
for that item or only requires review because of the cost of
the item. Many insurance companies have review criteria
based on dollar amount, for example, only reviewing items
that cost $1,000 or more. If your item is over the cutoff, ask

the vendor if they have models available under the review amount cutoff since prior approval may not be needed.

If you follow these steps and still find that your request has been denied by the insurance company, do you have any recourse? Absolutely yes.

Start by first understanding in detail the reason for the denial. Review the insurance denial letter with your doctor as well as a representative from the authorization department of insurance company. Once you and your doctor have understood the reason for the denial, the next step is for you, or even better, your doctor, to call the medical doctor at the insurance company to review your case. Keep a paper trail and document who replied from the insurance company, what they said, and keep all relevant records. A lot of denials are simply because the insurance company received incomplete information. In these instances, your doctor can clear it up with a simple conversation with the insurance company's medical director providing the missing information. Other times, you may not have met the insurance company criteria but may need to take additional measures or preliminary steps to meet the criteria. It is then just a matter of taking these steps and resubmitting the request. In the case of experimental procedures or services, it is helpful for the insurance company medical director to have a clear reason why other more standard treatments are not appropriate. For example, you may have tried all standard treatments unsuccessfully. It also important to emphasize what the medical consequences will be to you if you do not get the requested treatment, such as whether your health and quality of life will severely suffer. Your doctor should be able to back that up with specific information.

Failing the simple fix of discussing the case with the insurance company doctors, your case may need to be escalated. Most states and private insurances have an appeal process, where the information is resubmitted in writing to another individual or review board that looks at it with new eyes. For private insurance companies, the appeal process is usually listed in the denial letter or on the company website. In addition, with either an employer-provided insurance or an individual policy, you can opt for your state's appeals process. Often, these are handled through the state's insurance regulator, but if not, the agency should at least be able to tell you where to go. There are forty-four states that offer independent reviews, but it is important to check the state insurance website because each has its own rules. In the case of Medicare, there is a separate, federal appeals-review process that you can learn about at www.*Medicare.gov.*

Prepare for the appeal by ensuring that you follow the same tips outlined above for the insurance company discussion. Adding a brief cover letter addressing all the reasons outlined in the denial is also helpful. Your appeal may hinge on proving that your treatment is medically necessary. In that case, you will want to zero in on the medical guidelines and figure out why your request fits the criteria or why a medical exception should be made in your particular case. If the treatment you are getting is experimental, seek help from researchers who worked on the cutting-edge studies looking at the treatment. These doctors can help by reviewing your medical records and providing a backup letter on your behalf to support your own doctor. The support letter should prove that the research done in the field was well designed and executed and has yielded promising results. It also needs to show that there are no other established treatments that will help your particular case.

If you have been denied reimbursement for stay in a hospital or skilled nursing facility and it is the fault of the hospital or the doctor's decision making, then you should not be left holding the bag. Examples of this include a delay in providing you services while in the hospital, resulting in a longer hospitalization; or the care given was not complex enough to warrant being in the hospital. The facility may try to bill you for those days the insurance company denied. You should first try the steps outlined above with the insurance company. If this is not successful, then before agreeing to pay the hospital or skilled nursing facility, you should negotiate with the billing department and your doctor. If they are not agreeable, it may be important to consult a patient advocate service that can represent your case (see table 3). Many states have health insurance consumer advocates. The advocacy group Families USA offers a list of state resources available in their website.

Table 3: Patient Advocacy Organizations to Help with Insurance disputes

Patient Advocate Foundation
Hospitalbillreview.com
Healthproponent.com
Billadvocates.com
Healthchampion.net
Patientcare4u.com
Claims.org

In some instances, despite using all of the above methods for pursuing the outcome you want for your care, you may still not be successful with your preauthorization request. In these instances, if the service has not yet been provided, it may be an opportunity to rethink that option with your doctor. Is it really the only treatment option, or are there others that may be a good choice? The insurance company guidelines are actually derived from expert recommendations in the field and can sometimes act to protect an individual from unnecessary treatments. In other instances, you may decide that it is important to continue to press the issue. In these cases, there are three additional measures to consider.

1. **Go to the Top:** Consider appealing directly to the CEO of the insurance company. An article in the August 19, 2009 issue of the *Wall Street Journal*, "Taking Gripes Over Insurance to the Top Brass," details how a few consumers who had exhausted all other options successfully contacted top insurance company executives and had their issues resolved. The successful examples cited were not denied for medical issues, but rather administrative glitches. One case was because the insurance company mistakenly thought that the member had a preexisting condition. Another was because a data glitch from the employer incorrectly recorded the person's termination date, resulting in premature termination coverage through a former employer. Health-plan officials say they take complaint letters seriously, partly because they may reflect broader service breakdowns that need to be fixed. If you go this route, make sure you have already tried the traditional options already outlined. Be sure everything is thoroughly documented – including all your prior efforts, medical details of your case, dates of prior interactions with the insurance company and with which of

their employees. Be ready to provide any of these records that will back up your case if asked. The websites www. Consumerist.com and www.Emailnamefinder.com can help you figure out the e-mail addresses of executives.

2. **Publicize It:** The other strategy is to contact your local or even national media. Insurance companies and hospitals, like most other businesses, really dislike bad publicity. If you have a legitimate concern – a hospital is demanding payment even though the insurance denial is their fault, or your insurance is refusing to pay for a potentially life-saving treatment – the media may take it and run with it. Many local media stations have a local interest or consumer profile department and are looking for legitimate stories where consumers have been wronged. Closely related to this is sharing your experience on social media with consumer-opinion websites. Depending on your social media following, this may not make as much of a splash as news media exposure and may not resolve your issue. It can, however, potentially help others to avoid the pitfall you had with that particular company.

3. **Get Legal:** Finally, you may want to consider the legal option. If this dispute is over a large dollar amount, consider contacting an attorney to explain your problem and get advice. You can get a referral from a friend or contact your local bar association to find someone specializing in health-care disputes or consumer complaints. For smaller dollar amounts, small claims suits may be the better option. Dollar limits for small claims vary by state – from $1,500 in Kentucky to $25,000 in Tennessee – so check with your state court system.

Problems with Health Insurance – How to Report It

You may feel it necessary to report your insurance company for illegal or unethical practices. Start off by writing down names and date of any conversations you had for reference and keep all relevant records like denial letters and cancelled checks. For Medicare and Medicaid health plans, the *Beneficiary Ombudsman*, is an online government resource that explains how these and other government programs work and how to file a complaint or an appeal. People who are covered by private insurance should review the information they get when they enroll to find out who to contact when they have complaints. If you still do not feel that the issue has been resolved, you can elevate the dispute to the following:

1. **Your State Insurance Commissioner.** Almost all state insurance commissioners have health insurance complaint forms on their websites. They will follow up with some additional questions and may ask for supporting documents prior to contacting your health insurance company to discuss the issue. The commissioner's office will either close the investigation if no rules have been broken, or a specialist will work to address the issue.

2. **The Better Business Bureau (BBB).** Health insurance companies work hard to resolve complaints filed with the Better Business Bureau because they hurt sales. Many people check with the BBB before buying insurance.

Getting Help with Costs Insurance Doesn't Cover

Even with insurance, the cost of medical care can still be overwhelming. In addition to your premium, you are expected to pay the deductible, copayments, and, in some instances, co-insurance. Some insurance companies have caps on how much you will spend out of pocket while others have no limits. In addition, employers and insurance companies are now shifting more costs to consumers with high-deductible health plans. Many families are struggling to decide which bills they will pay and who in the family needs to see a doctor more.

There are actually many organizations that assist individuals with copays and deductibles. The catch is that they limit their focus to certain medical conditions. They provide help based on financial need, which requires the sharing of information about your financial situation. Many help with prescription drug costs. These organization are listed in the section "Getting Help with Your Medications." Below are examples of a few of the organizations that focus on copays and deductibles.

Caring Voice Coalition helps individuals affected by serious and chronic disorders and one of their programs, Vital Relief, provides need-based financial assistance limited to certain disorders or medical conditions.

The National Marrow Patient Assistance Program and Financial Assistance Fund: The Marrow Foundation is the fund-raising partner of the National Marrow Donor Program (NMDP). Funds from this program help individuals pay for searching the NMDP Registry and/or for some post-transplant costs. Applications for Patient Assistance Program funds must be submitted by an NMDP transplant center. Eligible individuals in need of bone marrow transplants may ask their transplant center coordinator to apply for one or both programs.

The Patient Access Network Foundation is a nonprofit 501(c)(3) organization dedicated to supporting the needs of patients that cannot access the treatments they need due to out-of-pocket health-care costs.

Patient Services Incorporated (PSI) is a nonprofit charitable organization that helps persons with specific chronic medical illnesses afford the high cost of health insurance premiums. Families are offered assistance based upon the severity of medical and financial need. In doing so, PSI offers a "safety net" for persons who "fall through the financial assistance cracks."

The HealthWell Foundation is a nonprofit that helps individuals with insurance who cannot afford their copayments, coinsurance, and premiums for important medical treatments. They support only certain medical conditions, so it is important to see if the one you are being treated for is on the list, which changes periodically based on funding availability.

Catastrophic Illness in Children Relief Fund. This fund covers expenses for the care of a child that insurance did not cover. Unlike charity care from the hospital, this fund covers both hospital expenses and doctor fees. Their online state application can start the process.

What If I Have No Health Insurance?

The percentage of people who have health insurance through their employers has been falling since 2000. This is leaving many individuals to pay for the steep costs of health insurance entirely on their own. If you are in this category, you need to consider other available options for coverage. Below are some alternatives for which you may qualify. These options are not available to everyone, but for those who meet the criteria, they offer a comprehensive coverage. In addition, this coverage may be available to people who already have a diagnosed medical condition, also called a preexisting condition.

Coverage Options for Those without Private Health Insurance

1. **Enroll in a public program.** Medicare offers free or reduced-fee medical insurance to seniors over age sixty-five and those with a recognized disability. Medicaid and the Children's Health Insurance Program does the same for children and/or families. Eligibility requirements vary from state to state, but in most states, uninsured children eighteen years old and younger whose family incomes are up to $46,000 per year (for a family of four) can qualify for either Medicaid or CHIP. To find out if you qualify, speak to a

hospital financial counselor in your area. Healthcare.gov's plan finder can also help you find more information. Either way, it is better to determine whether you qualify before you get sick. That way you can take advantage of preventive services too.

2. **Be a dependent on a family a group plan**. If you can be considered a dependent of a family member who has a job that offers dependent coverage, you can join their plan. Who can qualify as a dependent? Usually spouses, domestic partners or now, thanks to health reform, children up to age twenty-five. This is not usually an option for retiree-only plans and Medicare, which do not have the coverage option for adult children.

3. **Use COBRA**. COBRA is a federal program that allows you to continue the health insurance you had with your employer if you lose or leave your job. You have to pay the full amount of the premium that you and your employer paid, so a lot of times it can be very expensive. However, this may be cheaper than buying your own insurance or having to requalify for insurance if you or one of your dependents has a preexisting condition. COBRA coverage lasts only eighteen months.

4. **After COBRA runs out**. When COBRA coverage ends, there are two options for people who qualify. The first is a conversion plan that allows you to convert from the group employer plan to an individual plan. If you qualify for a conversion plan, you cannot be denied insurance because of your medical history. The other option is a HIPPA plan. To qualify for a HIPPA plan, you cannot have a lapse of more than sixty-three days in your coverage, and you must have had insurance through your employer for at least eighteen

months. For both these options, you have to pay the entire premium, so again, they are not cheap.

Seeking Care with No Insurance Coverage

If none of the above is an option for you and you find yourself with no health insurance, how do you afford medical care? Unfortunately, millions of Americans have had to face this situation. According to the Census Bureau, 48.6 million people, almost 1 in 5 Americans, have no health insurance. Getting medical care will vary depending on where you live and your age. However, there are certain resources that are common to most states or cities.

1. **Community Health Centers (CHCs):** CHCs often provide excellent basic medical care and sometimes dental and mental health services. Most areas have a community health center or a municipal, county, or city clinic system. Charges are based upon your ability to pay. They often have extended hours that can accommodate the schedule of working adults. CHCs also offer care for the whole family and often have programs that address the needs of the communities they serve. The websites of the National Association of Free and Charitable Clinics (NAFC) and the Health Resources and Services Administration provide online directories to find health centers and free clinics in your neighborhood.

2. **Mobile Clinics:** Mobile clinics are often a service that is provided by universities, city and state health departments, or nonprofit organizations. They often provide screenings

and care for high blood pressure, breast and prostate cancer, pregnancy and mental health. It is good to check the website of your local health department or nearby universities and hospitals to see if they sponsor a mobile clinic. While there are many nonprofits that sponsor mobile clinics, one that does so in many locations around the country is Remote Area Medical® (RAM). RAM operates mobile medical weekend expeditions where free dental, vision, and medical services are provided by volunteer licensed health practitioners on a first-come, first-served basis. The most frequent area visited is rural Appalachia, but RAM is expanding through affiliates to Oklahoma and California. The website ramusa.org provides a schedule of the towns they will be in for the year.

3. **Health fairs:** Like most mobile clinics, health fairs are good for screenings but not usually a permanent solution for health care. You can get free screenings and counseling for such conditions as hearing loss, high blood pressure, and high cholesterol. Some also offer free flu shots and vision screenings. The community groups who run them can often help connect you to resources if a health condition is detected.

4. **Free or reduced-price hospital care:** Many hospitals have programs for people who are struggling financially. Community Catalyst, a consumer advocacy group, has a website that describes relevant laws and policies in each state. For example, Maryland hospitals are required to tell a patient prior to discharge how they can apply for free and reduced-cost care. The best people to go to are the hospital billing office, social worker, or patient representative.

5. **Disease-specific programs:** Multiple programs exist that provide subsidized care for specific conditions, but you have to be eligible and follow very specific rules. They may cover many types of expenses, including medications, insurance copays, office visits, transportation, nutrition, medical supplies, child care, or respite care. Funding for these programs comes from both private and government organizations. Some programs are national in scope, while others are limited to people in specific states. Most have some type of eligibility requirements, usually financial ones. For example, the federally funded Breast and Cervical Cancer Treatment Program will pay for all disease-specific treatment for women with low incomes. However, qualifying requires that your condition was diagnosed at one of the program's approved screening centers. If you received a diagnosis elsewhere, you're not eligible. Needymeds. org, a website run by a nonprofit group, lists a number of financial-assistance programs for specific diseases, covering everything from camps and scholarships to respite care, in an easy-to-search format.

6. **Teaching dental clinics:** these clinics, called predoctoral dental clinics, are where young dentists and dental hygienists are trained. Fees are much lower than those of practicing dentists. The care is provided by students closely supervised by a faculty member and includes most types of minor and major dental procedures.

7. **Comparison shop:** there are an increasing number of websites, such as HealthcareBlueBook.com, that let consumers see the prices of medically related services, anything from breast reduction surgery to a physician

office visit. One thing that is readily apparent is the wide price discrepancies for a given procedure or service. For example, California hospitals charge anywhere from $1,529 to $182,955, with a median cost of $33,611, for routine appendicitis. OutOfPocket.com provides a comparison pricing service that also allows visitors to post the prices they paid for services, and it then pulls in payment data from private insurers and Medicare available on other websites. There is also education about what certain tests and procedures are as well as how to get the best rates at any given facility. Knowing when there are wide price disparities can help you negotiate a reasonable rate. It is important to remember, though, that these sites do not offer quality data, so there is no way yet, without extra research, to determine the best "deal" – the best quality service for the lowest price.

What Not to Do:

If you do not have insurance, accessing emergency department (ED) care can be the most expensive option for health care. It is true that EDs cannot turn you away. But their obligation is to stabilize you, not comprehensively address your ailment. For the highly skilled, convenient, twenty-four-hour service of an emergency department, you will receive a large bill afterward, and the hospital might be very aggressive about trying to collect payment. If you think you have a true emergency, by all means use this resource. However, if your condition is not an emergency, it is better to be seen in a city clinic or an urgent care center. One resource to help determine if you have a true emergency is iTriage. com, which has a mobile app for smartphones developed to help consumers figure where they should go for treatment. Another might be the twenty-four-hour nurse line of your health insurance company.

Paying for Medical Bills Once They Are Incurred

Sometimes, even if we do not want to, we have to go to a hospital unexpectedly. Predictably, this can result in massive hospital bills. But you are not totally without options. There are also options for payment available to you. What not to do? Ignore the bill. Your first step after you get treatment should be to get a detailed bill to look for procedures and items that you did not actually receive. Since bills can be hard to read, the hospital billing office, where you can get a bill copy, can help to walk you through each line. Nonprofit patient advocate organizations like *Patient Advocate Foundation* or claims consultants can help, although for-profit ones will charge you for the advice.

After inaccurate charges are removed, next address the rest of the bill. Ask the billing office staff if there is a charity department. Most, if not all, hospitals have a one. The charity department can set a sliding scale for payment or even write off a certain percentage of the charges. Nonprofit hospitals often receive outside funding to cover care to those who cannot afford it. To apply for charity care or receive payment help, you must be under a certain income level, report your household dependents and your income, and provide proof of identity and residency.

The next step is to negotiate. You can negotiate reduced hospital fees even if your income is too high to qualify for charity care. It is important to remember, though, that charity care programs only cover hospital expenses, not doctors' fees. But you can take the same approach to individual doctor fees – negotiate! For the doctor or hospital, negotiating a reduced fee that gets paid is better than receiving no payment at all for a full bill. Consider this – if a collection agency takes the case, they may charge 10 to 50 percent of the debt. So many providers and hospitals will discount the bill at least this much in order to get payment up front. In addition, many consumers do not realize that insurance companies do not pay the full rate for doctor services or hospital fees. Doctors and hospitals, since they accept a reduced payment from insurance companies, will likely be open to accepting a lower rate for self-pay individuals. The key is to ask.

Once a rate is negotiated or a sliding fee set, the most important thing to do is to continue to pay something toward the debt every month. Doing this inspires confidence that you are making an effort to resolve the debt. As a result, the institution or doctor's office is unlikely to turn the debt over to a collection agency and thereby affect your credit.

Special Resources for Those without Insurance

Just as there are resources to help insured individuals with bills they cannot pay, there are similar organizations to help those without any health insurance.

1. **Funds for Children**: Each state has designated resources available for children from families without insurance called the Catastrophic Illness in Children Relief Fund. Unlike charity care from the hospital, this fund covers both hospital

expenses and doctor fees. The state application can be found online.

2. **Federal Programs for Seniors**: The National Council on Aging lets you as a senior know the federal programs for which you are eligible. The interactive website takes you through a series of questions to identify benefit programs that can help you pay for medications, health care, food, utilities, and more.

3. **Programs for Those with Disability:** The federal government has a website offering comprehensive information on programs and services for individuals with disability in communities nationwide. The site links to more than fourteen resources from federal, state and local government agencies, academic institutions, and nonprofits.

4. **Programs Sponsored by Religious and Social Service Organizations**: Local social service agencies or religious groups may have emergency funds for emergency hospital bills. Try United Way, Salvation Army, Goodwill, or a church, synagogue, or mosque for help. A great local resource for finding the right social service agency is the 2-1-1 system. It provides free and confidential referral information on health care, counseling, and other related needs.

No Need to Skip Your Meds

Affording medications may be an ongoing issue if you have a chronic illness. Many people skip taking medicines in order to pay for other bills. They may not know that there are ways to keep their medication costs low as well as resources to help with prescription payment. Let us start with ways to keep costs down.

1. **Stick with your health plan's list of covered prescription drugs.** This list is also known as a formulary. If your doctor only prescribes medications from the formulary, you will not have to pay the full cost for an expensive name-brand medicine. Closely related to this is your doctor first trying the least expensive option, like a generic, and only going to the more expensive choice if the first does not provide the result you want.

2. **Bargain Shop:** Mail-order pharmacies often provide discounts on medications that are needed on a recurring basis. Insurance companies often offer discounts and incentives for getting your medications from their affiliated mail-order pharmacies. For brick-and-mortar pharmacies, make sure to comparison shop at more than one pharmacy. The list of pharmacies that offer $4 generic medications continues to grow – Kroger, Walmart, Target – and as long as you are willing to purchase generic, you can take advantage of these discounts.

3. **Know what discounts are available from your insurance company** – Insurance companies offer discount incentives for choosing generics. In addition, some insurance companies offer coaching programs with no or reduced medication copays in exchange for participation. Here is how it works. If you agree to talk with a nurse, you get individualized coaching for your health condition and get medications for that condition with no copay. The catch is you have to have one of the conditions – usually diabetes,

high blood pressure, or heart disease – covered by these programs.

If your medication cost remains high despite these options, there is still assistance available from a variety of organizations designed to assist with medication purchases. Even with insurance, copays for some medications can be between $300 and $3,000 per month, so financial assistance for many is a necessity.

Copay Relief: The Patient Advocate Foundation (PAF) Co-Pay Relief Program (CPR) currently assists insured patients who are financially and medically qualified and are being treated for specific cancers, cancer-related conditions, osteoporosis, pain, hepatitis C, and rheumatoid arthritis. The full list can be found on their website.

The Chronic Disease Fund covers selected drugs for cancers and other chronic diseases like multiple sclerosis and Crohn's disease.

Partnership for Prescription Assistance (PPARX): PPARX is a coalition of America's pharmaceutical companies, health-care providers, patient advocacy organizations, and community groups that helps qualifying patients without prescription drug coverage get free or low-cost medicines. They match you with an appropriate public or private program based on the medication(s) you need. The PPARX website lists resources for assistance by disease, program, and region. Program participants may get their medications for free or nearly free.

Pharmaceutical Company Patient Assistance Programs (PAPs) offer free medications for a variety of conditions to people with low incomes who do not qualify for any other assistance programs. To know if this can benefit you, find out what drug company manufactures your medication and call or go their website to see if they have a patient assistance program for your medication. Different company programs have different eligibility criteria. Most, though, are based on the Federal Poverty Level (FPL) designation, which can be calculated based on family or household size. Unless otherwise stated, companies ask for verification of income, usually in the form of a federal income tax return. Even if you do not meet the requirements, you should always apply for an exception.

Faith Community Pharmacy: The Faith Community Pharmacy is a 501(c)(3) nonprofit organization created to provide free prescription medication to residents of Northern Kentucky in need. Some prescription medications are donated by area physician's and drug manufacturers. Other medications must be purchased, such as insulin and generic medications. Costs are kept to a minimum by using volunteers and intern students from the University of Cincinnati College of Pharmacy.

The **NeedyMeds Drug Discount Card** provides a card that allows for up to 80 percent off the price of your prescription medications. The card is available to anyone free of charge on their website. It can be used by those without insurance and by those who decide not to use their insurance – for example, if the drug is not covered under your plan, the copay or deductible is high, the cap has been reached, or if you are in the Medicare "donut hole." In addition to prescription medications, it can also be used for over-the-counter medications and medical supplies if written on a prescription pad by your doctor. The card is accepted at over sixty-two thousand pharmacies, including popular chains like Walmart, CVS, Walgreens, and Rite Aid.

The Together Rx Access® Card is a discount card sponsored by several pharmaceutical companies that anyone can use to get savings on prescriptions at most pharmacies. It covers over three hundred brand-name prescription medicines and products and some generic products. Medicines in the program include those used to treat high cholesterol, diabetes, depression, asthma, and many other common conditions. You can download it from their website.

The **CancerCare Co-Payment Assistance Foundation** is a nonprofit organization that helps individuals who cannot afford their insurance copayments to cover the cost of medications for treating cancer. The foundation has a list of about eight cancer types which they provide financial assistance in paying for medications to treat those specific cancers and the cost of administering them.

Paying for Complementary and Alternative Care

Spending on Complementary and Alternative Medicine (CAM) treatments is over a $33 million industry in the U.S. and growing. These therapies are paid for largely out of pocket. Private health insurance plans may offer coverage of certain CAM therapies, usually chiropractic, acupuncture, and massage. Overall, however, coverage of CAM therapies is very limited. One factor is a lack of scientific evidence regarding the effectiveness of CAM therapies. However, slowly, more insurance companies and managed care organizations – like BCBS of Texas, Anthem, and the University of Pittsburgh Medical Center Health Plan – are offering coverage of CAM therapies shown to be safe and effective.

If you are planning to use a CAM service, find out about payment before you begin treatment. If you have insurance, start off finding out if the service you want is covered and what kind of restrictions may apply. Keep records about all contacts you have with the insurance company, including notes on calls and copies of bills, claims, and letters as usual, just in case a dispute arises about a claim. Up-front questions you need to ask of your insurance company include:

- Is there is a higher deductible and/or copayment than for conventional care?
- Do you need prior approval for your payment request from the insurance company before starting care?
- Do you need a referral from your primary-care physician?
- Do you have to stay within an approved network of providers?

- Are there are limits on the number of visits or the annual dollar amount paid?

Some insurance companies offer what are called CAM "riders" that are an add-on to your policy. Riders can be purchased at an additional cost, but will provide coverage for certain CAM therapies. Keep in mind that if you have either a "flexible spending account" or a "health savings account" you can use these funds to pay for CAM therapy. If your insurance company covers CAM or you have purchased a rider, one question to ask the provider is whether they submit the claim, or do they expect you to pay up front and submit the claim yourself.

For those whose visits insurance does not cover, your next step is to know about the provider's costs.

- Costs: What does the first appointment cost? What do follow-up appointments cost? How many appointments am I likely to need? Are there any additional costs (e.g., tests, equipment, supplements)?
- Payment options: If you are unable to pay the full fee for each visit, you need to ask the provider – Can you arrange a payment plan over time? Do you offer a sliding-scale fee (i.e., fees based on income and ability to pay)?

Finally, remember like other health expenses, some CAM expenses may be tax deductible. The IRS allows taxpayers to deduct medical expenses for acupuncture, chiropractic care, and osteopathic care.

Provider-Specific Payment Situations and Discounts

There are certain discounts and payment options available only with specific types of therapies. Knowing about these options may allow you to fit these types of therapies into your budget.

Acupuncture Clinics – a little known resource for affordable acupuncture care is through community acupuncture clinics. In these settings, acupuncture is practiced in a group, with one practitioner treating several patients at a time, rather than in a one-on-one setting. Community-style clinics run on a sliding scale, $20-$40 per session, in contrast to a private session of $90 or more. These clinics exist in order to make acupuncture more affordable and accessible to the general population.

Massage – call local massage therapy schools to find out if the students being trained provide discounted massages.

Chiropractic Doctors – if you can afford it, see if your chiropractor offers a paid-in-advance discount. This payment option involves prepaying an entire prescribed regimen or paying in advance for a certain number of sessions. Typically, the chiropractor will reduce the fees and potentially add extra services at no additional cost.

Integrative Medicine Doctors – we discussed earlier how integrative medicine combines conventional western medicine with alternative therapies. Often, because these doctors are recognized by insurance companies as conventional practitioners, part or all of their consultation will be reimbursed. Often, though, they will have you pay up front and submit the paperwork for reimbursement directly to your insurance company. It is still a way to have some or most of your visit cost covered.

Takeaway Checklist

Buying Insurance

☐ Know if you are selecting an indemnity plan, managed care plan (HMO, POS, PPO), or consumer-driven high-deductible health plan with an HRA or HSA.

☐ Know the costs associated – the premium, deductible, copay, coinsurance; also know if there are caps set on what you will have to spend out of pocket.

☐ Know what services the plan covers – is it comprehensive enough for you needs?

☐ Does the plan have the flexibility you need?

☐ Stick to the kinds of high-quality health plans that can be found on the Healthcare.gov website and enquire with the Better Business Bureau and the State Insurance Commissioner's office to ensure no complaints have been lodged against them.

Managing Requests for Health Insurance Companies to Cover Medical Services for You

☐ Know your insurance company Plan Description document well so that you will know the insurance benefits that are covered and those which are not

☐ Make sure you communicate all relevant information to your doctor before they submit your request for a particular service.

☐ Make sure your doctor submits the precertification request at least three weeks in advance of an elective procedure.

☐ Your doctor can get a copy of the detailed guidelines that explain the insurance company criteria for pre-certification in order to prepare to submit the request for coverage.

If your request is not honored:

☐ Ask your doctor to call the medical doctor at the insurance company to review your case.

☐ Keep a paper trail and document who replied from the insurance company and what they said.

☐ Take any steps recommended and resubmit the necessary documentation with the request.

☐ Know your insurance companies appeal process, the state's appeals process, or the federal appeals-review process if it is for Medicare.

☐ Add a brief cover letter addressing all the reasons outlined in the denial.

☐ If your claim still is denied after appeal, reevaluate if your request it is truly the best option for your health with a second opinion; if so, other avenues for recourse include the insurance company leadership, the media, or a lawyer.

☐ Report unfair insurance practices to the state health commissioner or the Better Business Bureau.

Coverage Options for Those without Health Insurance

☐ Enroll in a public program like Medicare, Medicaid, and the Children's Health Insurance Program with information from a clinic or hospital financial counselor, or on Healthcare. gov's plan finder.

☐ Become a dependent on a family a group plan if you are a spouse, domestic partner, or child under age twenty-six.

☐ Use COBRA benefits from prior coverage.

☐ See if you qualify for a conversion plan or a HIPPA plan after COBRA runs out.

Paying for Medical Bills Once They Are Incurred

☐ Get a detailed copy of the bill from the hospital billing office to look for procedures and items that you did not actually receive.

☐ Ask the billing office staff if there is a charity department.

☐ Negotiate write-offs or reduced hospital fees with the hospital and with the doctor's office.

☐ Continue to pay something toward the debt every month.

Affording Medications By Keeping Costs Down

☐ Stick with your health plan's list of covered prescription drugs.

☐ Mail-order pharmacies provide discounts on medications that are needed on a recurring basis. Use pharmacies that offer $4 generic medications if you have a generic brand on their list.

☐ Find out what discounts are available from your insurance company.

☐ Double your medicine dose and then take half – check with your pharmacist or doctor to see if this can be done safely with your medicine.

☐ See if copay assistance is available for the medications you take.

Paying for Complementary and Alternative Care

If you have health insurance, find out from your health plan if

☐ they offer coverage for the CAM therapies you want;

☐ there is a higher deductible and/or copayment than for conventional care;

☐ you need prior approval for your payment request from the insurance company before starting care;

☐ you need a referral from your primary-care physician;

☐ you have to stay within an approved network of providers;

☐ there are limits on the number of visits or the annual dollar amount paid

☐ you can purchase a CAM "rider" as an add-on to your policy

☐ you can use your funds from your flexible spending account *or* health savings account.

If you will not be covered by insurance or do not have insurance, inquire about the following:

☐ What does the first appointment cost? What do follow-up appointments cost? How many appointments am I likely to need? Are there any additional costs?

☐ What are the payment options? Is there a payment plan, sliding-scale fee, discount for paying up front?

☐ Check with the IRS to see if your CAM expenses are tax deductible.

☐ For lower cost acupuncture, see if there is a community acupuncture clinic in your area.

☐ For lower cost massage, call local massage therapy schools.

Conclusion

As I see it, every day you do one of two things:
build health or produce disease in yourself.

– Adelle Davis

B EING HIT WITH an unexpected diagnosis often takes the wind out of our sails. But it is also a time to reevaluate, regroup, and formulate an approach as an active participant in your health. To that end, we have covered a lot of ground to help you prepare for this more empowered role. We started with your lifestyle choices, built with your buddy network, and expanded out to working with the health-care team you choose as your partner. We also looked at strategies for getting the best care through first caring for yourself; finding the best doctors, complementary practitioners, hospitals, and clinical trials; and finally, how to not go broke while doing so.

Our health-care system is changing at an unprecedented rate. There are now more options coming on to the horizon for getting health insurance coverage. These coverage options will allow many more people to access health care. In addition, more treatment options are available with complementary and alternative practitioners practicing alongside conventional doctors. The conventional health-care system is becoming more focused around the patients' needs with Patient-Centered Medical Homes. And finally, whole new ways of approaching medical problems are being developed – from nanomedicine to stem cell therapies. But no matter what these changes bring, being an educated health-care consumer allows you to evaluate whether something is for you. You can participate with your health-care provider in safeguarding your health.

Health is a journey, and the net effect of our lives each day is to take a step closer toward it or away from it. As you move forward on your journey, you can use this book as a guide to make sure you are equipped to handle the wide variety of health-care situations that are a part of this journey. Together with your health-care partners, you will be able to put together an integrated plan that enables you to take more steps forward every day.

Selected Bibliography

Chapter 2

1. Kohn, L. T., Corrigan, J., & Donaldson, M. S. (2000). *To err is human: Building a safer health system.* Washington, DC: National Academy Press.
2. Bodenheimer T., Wagner E.H., & Grumbach K. (2002, October 22). Improving primary care for patients with chronic illness: the chronic care model, Part 2. 1909-14.
3. Osborn R. (April/June 2012). "International Perspectives on Patient Engagement: Results from the 2011 Commonwealth

Fund Survey." *Journal of Ambulatory Care Management, April/ June 2012*, 118-28.

4. Katon W (2002). Impact of major depression on chronic medical illness. *Journal of Psychosomatic Research 53 (2002) 859-863*, 859-863.

5. Dimatteo, M.R., Lepper, H.S., & Crogan, T.W. (2000). Depression is a risk factor for noncompliance with medical treatment: meta-analysis of the effects of anxiety and depression on patient adherence. *Arch Intern Med*, 160: 2101-2107.

6. Arnstein P. (2002). From chronic pain patient to peer: Benefits and risks of volunteering. *Pain Management Nursing. 3(3)*, 84-103.

7. Helmes E. (2007). Differences between Older Adult Volunteers and Non-volunteers in Depression and Self-efficacy. *Australian Journal on Volunteering. 12(12)*, 30-36.

8. Mccoubrie R. (2006). Is there a correlation between spirituality and anxiety and depression in patients with advanced cancer? *Supportive Care in Cancer, 14(4)*, 379-385.

Chapter 3

1. Nicklas B.J. (2004). Diet-induced weight loss, exercise, and chronic inflammation in older, obese adults: a randomized controlled clinical trial. *American Journal of Clinical Nutrition, 79(4)*, 544-551.

2. Sikaris K.A. (2004). The Clinical Biochemistry of Obesity. *Clin Biochem Review, 25(3)*, 165-181.

3. McNulty A.L. (2011). The effects of adipokines on cartilage and meniscus catabolism. *Connective Tissue Research, 52(6)*, 523-33.

4. O'Rourke L. (2002). Glucose-dependent regulation of cholesterol ester metabolism in macrophages by insulin and leptin. *Journal of Biological Chemistry. 277,* 42557-42562.

5. Yudkin J.S. (2000). Inflammation, obesity, stress and coronary heart disease: is interleukin-6 the link? *Atherosclerosis, 148,* 209-214.

6. Rabe K.(2008). Adipokines and Insulin Resistance. *Mol Med. 11(12),* 741-751.

7. Ford E.S. (1997). Weight change and diabetes incidence: findings from a national cohort of US adults. *Am J Epidemiol, 146(3),* 214-22.

8. Colditz G.A. (1990). Weight as a risk factor for clinical diabetes in women. *Am J Epidemiol. "132(3)",* 501-13.

9. Yamauchi T. (2002). Adiponectin stimulates glucose utilization and fatty-acid oxidation by activating AMP-activated protein kinase. *Nature Medicine, 8,* 1288-1295.

10. Pischon T. (2004). Plasma adiponectin levels and risk of myocardial infarction in men. *Journal of American Medical Association, 291,* 1730-1737.

Chapter 4

1. Preamble to the Constitution of the World Health Organization as adopted by the International Health Conference, New York, 19-22 June, 1946; signed on 22 July 1946 by the representatives of 61 States (Official Records of

the World Health Organization, no. 2, p. 100) and entered into force on 7 April 1948.

2. Sullivan, K. (2012, August, 1). *Welcome to sunlightd.org.* SunlightandVitaminD.org. Retrieved August 30, 2012, from http://www.sunlightandvitamind.org.

3. Vitamin D Council. (2012, July, 9).*Vitamin D deficiency: A Global Epidemic.* VitaminDcouncil.org. Retrieved August 5, 2012, from http://www.vitamindcouncil.org/about-vitamin-d/vitamin -d-deficiency

4. *Vitamin D and your health: Breaking old rules, raising new hopes.* (2007, February). Retrieved March 25, 2012, from http:// www.health.harvard.edu/newsweek/vitamin-d-and-your-health.htm.

5. Skae, T. (2008, March 28). The Healing Benefits of Sunlight and Vitamin D. Retrieved November 22, 2011, from http:// www.naturalnews.com.

6. Lappe J.P. (2007). Vitamin D and calcium supplementation reduces cancer risk: results of a randomized trial. *Am J Clinical Nutrition,85(6)*, 1586-91.

7. Henendez C. (2001). Retinoic acid and Vitamin D(3) powerfully inhibit in vitro leptin secretion by human adipose tissue. *J Endocrinol, 170(2)*, 435-31.

8. McMichael A.J. (2001). Multiple sclerosis and ultraviolet radiation: time to shed more light. *Neuroepidemiology2, 0(3)*, 165-7.

9. Wortsman J (2000). Decreased bioavailability of Vitamin D in obesity. *Am J Clinical Nutrition, 72(3)*, 690-3.

10. Koren D., Levitt Katz L.E., Brar P.C., Gallagher P.R., Berkowitz R.I., Brooks L.J. Sleep architecture and glucose

and insulin homeostasis in obese adolescents. Diabetes Care, 2011 Nov 34(11):2442-7.

11. Boergres J. (2007). Child sleep disorders: Associations with parental sleep duration and daytime sleepiness. *Journal of Family Psychology*, *21*, 88-94.

12. Gregory A.M. (2012). Sleep, emotional and behavioral difficulties in children and adolescents. *Sleep Medicine Reviews*, *16*, 129-136.

13. Mindell J.A. (2011). Give children and adolescents the gift of a good night's sleep: a call to action. *Sleep Medicine, 12*, 203-204.

14. 2013 Sleep in America®Poll Task Force. (2013, March 4). 2013 *Sleep in America®*. National Sleep Foundation. Retrieved March 25, 2013, at http://www.sleepfoundation.org.

15. Archie Comics. (1973).Archie's Love Scene Disk 106:537, Dy1:Archi3.Txt. Archie Enterprises. Old Tappan, NJ: Fleming Revell Co. Retrieved on October 11, 2012 from http://www.soc.cornell.edu/hayes-lexical-analysis/CornellCorpus2000/comics/ARCHIE03.ASC

16. Brown WJ (2007). Updating the evidence on physical activity and health in women. *Am J Prev Med., 33(5)*, 404-411.

17. Gleeson M (2007). Immune function in sport and exercise. *J Appl Physiol. 103(2)*, 693-9.

18. Physical Activity Guidelines. (2008). HHS.gov. Retrieved March 25, 2013, from www.hhs.gov

19. Wang J. (2007). Short term meditation training improves attention and self regulation. *Proceedings of the National Academy of Sciences, 104(43)*, 17152-17156.

20. Kabat-Zinn, J. (1990). *Full Catastrophe Living: Using the Wisdom of Your Body and Mind to Face Stress, Pain and Illness.* New York, NY: Delacorte Press.

21. Astin, John A et al. "Meditation." In Donald Novey *(Ed.) Clinician's Complete Reference to Complementary and Alternative Medicine.* St. Louis, MO: Mosby, 2000.

22. Wikipedia (2012, April 18) Cyberchondria. Wikipedia.com. *Retrieved January, 12, 2013 from http://en.wikipedia.org/wiki/ Cyberchondria.*

23. Medline Plus.(2013, March 14). Evaluating Health Information. MedlinePlus – *Health Information from the National Library of Medicine.* Retrieved April 12, 2013, from http://www.nlm. nih.gov/medlineplus/evaluatinghealthinformation.html

24. Densen P. (2011). Challenges and Opportunities Facing Medical Education. *Trans Am Clin Climatol Assoc., 122*, 48-58.

25. Barnes L. (2004). Social Resources and Cognitive Decline in a Population of Older African Americans and Whites. *Neurology, 63*, 2322-26.

26. Brummett H. (2001). Characteristics of Socially Isolated Patients with Coronary Artery Disease Who are at Elevated Risk for Mortality. *Psychosmatic Medicine, 63*, 67-272.

27. Cohen S. (1997). Social Ties and Susceptibility to the Common Cold. *Journal of American Medical Association, 277*, 1940-44.

28. Heikkinen L. (2004). Depressive Symptoms in Late Life: A 10-Year Follow-Up. *Archives of Gerontology and Geriatrics, 38*, 239-50.

29. House J.S. (2001). Social Isolation Kills, But How and Why? *Psychosomatic Medicine, 63*, 273-74.

30. Pressman S.D. (2005). Loneliness, Social Network Size, and Immune Response to Influenza Vaccination in College Freshmen. *Health Psychology, 24*, 297-306.

31. Seeman T.E. (2000). Health Promoting Effects of Friends and Family on Health Outcomes in Older Adults. *American Journal of Health Promotion, 64*, 234-40.

32. Wilson R.S. (2007). Loneliness and Risk of Alzheimer Disease. *Archives of General Psychiatry, 64*, 234-40.

33. Uchino B.N. (1996). The Relationship Between Social Support and Physiological Processes: A Review with Emphasis on Underlying Mechanisms and Implications for Health. *Psychological Bulletin, 119*, 488-531.

34. Blue, L. (2010, July 28). *Recipe for Longevity: No Smoking, Lots of Friends.* Time.com. Retrieved October 6, 2012, from http://www.time.com.

35. Engel KG (2009). Patient Comprehension of Emergency Department Care and Instructions: Are Patients Aware of When They Do Not Understand? *Ann Emerg Med.,53*, 454-461.

Chapter 5

1. Pearson, J. (1985). *Is There A Doctor in the House? A Guide to Choosing a Physician.* Medicine-in-Motion.com. Retrieved July 2, 2012 from *http://www.medicine-in-motion.com.*

2. American College of Physicians (2008). *How Is a Shortage of Primary Care Physicians Affecting the Quality and Cost of Medical Care?* (White Paper) Philadelphia: American College of Physicians. Available from American College of

Physicians, 190 N. Independence Mall West, Philadelphia, PA 19106.

3. Flanagan L. (1998). Practitioners: Growing Competition for Family Physicians? Changes in state laws and strong consumer support make a discussion of the role of independent nurse practitioners unavoidable. *Fam Pract Manag, 5(9)*, 34-43.

4. Lesho E.P. (1999). "An overview of osteopathic medicine." *Archives of Family Medicine, 8(6)*, 477-84.

5. Licciardone J. (2002). Patient satisfaction and clinical outcomes associated with osteopathic manipulative treatment. *The Journal of the American Osteopathic Association, 102(1)*, 12-20.

6. National Center for Complementary and Alternative Medicine. (2012, April, 09). Naturopathy: An Introduction. Nccam.nih.gov. Retrieved July 25, 2012, from http://nccam.nih.gov/health/naturopathy/naturopathyintro.htm#hed5.

7. Herman P.M. (2008). Cost-effectiveness of naturopathic care for chronic low back pain. *Alternative Therapies in Health and Medicine, 14(2)*, 32-39.

8. Boons H.S. (2004). Practice patterns of naturopathic physicians: results from a random survey of licensed practitioners in two US States. *BMC Complement Altern Med., 20(4)*, 14.

9. Ehrlich, S. (2011, October, 12). *Naturopathy: Overview.* Umm.edu. Retrieved February 13, 2012 from http://www.umm.edu/altmed/articles/naturopathy-000356.htm#ixzz1sSFckZPk

10. Atwood K.C. (2003). Naturopathy: a critical appraisal. *Med Gen Med.,5(4)*, 39.

11. Jagtenberg T. (2006). Evidence-based medicine and naturopathy. *J Altern Complement Med, 12(3)*, 323-328.

12. Pizzorno J.E. (2005). Naturopathic medicine – a 10-year perspective (from a 35-year view). *Altern Ther Health Med,11(2)*, 24-26.

13. Smith M.J. (2002). Naturopathy. *Med Clin North Am, 86(1)*, 173-184.

14. Steven, D. (2011, October, 2). *Chiropractic: Overview.* Umm.edu. Retrieved February 16, 2012, from http://www.umm.edu/altmed/articles/chiropractic-000350.htm#ixzz1sXhDUIFu

15. Bishop PB (2010). The Chiropractic Hospital-based Interventions Research Outcomes (CHIRO) Study: a randomized controlled trial on the effectiveness of clinical practice guidelines in the medical and chiropractic management of patients with acute mechanical low back pain. *Spine Journal, 10*, 1055-1064.

16. Kasprak, J. (2010, August, 03). *Homeopathic Licensure.* Cga.ct.gov. Retrieved February 1, 2013, from http://www.cga.ct.gov/2010/rpt/2010-R-0315.htm

17. Steven, D. (2011, December, 14). *NMD. Acupuncture: Overview.* Umm.edu. Retrieved February 26, 2012, from http://www.umm.edu/altmed/articles/acupuncture-000345.htm#ixzz1sY15vm5s

18. Tyme, L.Ac.(2001). Student Manual on the Fundamentals of Traditional Oriental Medicine. La Mesa, CA: Living Earth Enterprises.

19. Ross J. (1995). Acupuncture Point Combinations: *The Key to Clinical Success. Churchill Livingstone. Philadelphia, PA : Churchill Livingstone.*

20. Steven, D (2011, October, 02). *Ayurveda: Overview.* Umm. edu Retrieved February 16, 2012, from http://www.umm. edu/altmed/articles/ayurveda-000348.htm#ixzz1sajD1iFV

21. World Health Organization. (2010). Benchmarks for training in traditional, complementary and alternative medicine: benchmarks for training in Ayurveda. Geneva, Switzerland: World Health Organization, WHO Press.

22. Park J. (2005). Ayurvedic Medicine for Rheumatoid Arthritis: A Systematic Review. *Seminars in Arthritis and Rheumatism, 34(5),* 705-713.

23. *National Center for Complementary and Alternative Medicine* (NCCAM) (2012, January 18). Ayurvedic Medicine. Nccam. nih.gov. Retrieved March 2, 2012, from 4 http://nccam.nih. gov/health/ayurveda.

24. Saper, R. B., Phillips, R. S. et al. (2008). *"Lead, Mercury, and Arsenic in US – and Indian-manufactured Ayurvedic Medicines Sold via the Internet." Journal of the American Medical Association* **300** (8): 915-23. Retrieved March 2, 2012, from http//www. ncbi.nlm.nih.gov/pmc/articles/PMC2755247/.

25. Valiathan, M. S. (2006). *"Ayurveda: Putting the House in Order." Current Science (Indian Academy of Sciences)* **90** (1): 5-6. Retrieved March 2, 2012, from *http://www.ias.ac.in/currsci/ jan102006/contents.htm.*

26. Epp A, et al.(2009) *Applications of individual cognitive-behavioral therapy to specific disorders: Efficacy and indications.* In: G.O.Gabbard, Textbook of Psychotherapeutic Treatments. Arlington, VA: American Psychiatric Publishing. Retrieved July 15, 2010 from http://www.psychiatryonline.com

27. National Association of Cognitive-Behavioral Therapists. "What Is Cognitive Behavioral Therapy?" NACBT.org.

Retrieved March 2, 2012, from http://www.nacbt.org/whatiscbt.htm.

28. Krenke K. (2000). Cognitive-Behavioral Therapy for Somatization and Symptom Syndromes: A Critical Review of Controlled Clinical Trials. *Psychother Psychosom*, 69, 205-215.

29. Patel K.C., Gross A., Graham N., Goldsmith C.H., Ezzo J., Morien A., Peloso P.M.J.(2012, September 12). Massage for mechanical neck disorders. Cochrane Database of Systematic Reviews, 2012, Issue 9. Art. No.: CD004871. DOI: 10.1002/14651858.CD004871.pub4.

30. Ezzo J., Donner T., Nickols, D, & Cox M. (2001). Is Massage Useful in the Management of Diabetes? A Systematic Review. Diabetes Spectrum, 14(4) 218-224.

31. Wilkinson S. (2008). Massage for symptom relief in patients with cancer: systematic review. *J Adv Nurs, 63(5)*, 430-439.

32. Vickers A., Ohlsson A., Lacy J.B., Horsley A. (2000). Massage for promoting growth and development in low birth-weight infants. Cochrane Database Syst Rev. 2004;(2):CD000390.

33. Viggo, H.S. et al. (2006). Massage and touch for dementia. Cochrane Database of Systematic Reviews, 2006 Oct 18;(4):CD004989.

34. Fulran A.D. Brosseau L., Imamura M., Irvin E. (2008). Massage for low-back pain. Cochrane Database Syst Rev. 2002;(2):CD001929.

35. Steven, E.D (2011, December, 14). *Massage: Overview*. Umm. edu. Retrieved April 21, 2012, from http://www.umm.edu/altmed/articles/massage-000354.htm#ixzz1siZP2qmL

36. Robertson D. (2009). Which Forms of Hypnotherapy are Evidence-Based? Hypnotherapy as Empirically-Supported Treatment (EST). Reprinted from *The Hypnotherapy Journal*

Spring 2009. Retrieved on April 21, 2012 from http://www. nwmedicalhypnosis.com.

37. Chambless D.L. et al. (1998). Update on empirically validated therapies II. *Clin Psychol.*, *51*, 3-16.

38. Wark D.M (2008). What we can do with hypnosis: a brief note. Am J Clin Hypnosis, 51(1), 29-36. DOI:10.1080/00029 157.2008.10401640

39. Steven, E.D (2011, September 6). *Hypnotherapy: Overview.* Umm.edu. Retrieved April 23, 2012, from http://www.umm. edu/altmed/articles/hypnotherapy-000353.htm#ixzz1slzI71ri

40. HHS/ACF/ACYF/HSB. (2002). What Are the Differences Between a Registered Dietitian (RD) and a Nutritionist? Early Head Start Tip Sheet No. 7. Eclkc.ohs.acf.hhs.gov Retrieved June 22, 2013 from http://eclkc.ohs.acf.hhs.gov/ hslc/tta-system/health/Health/nutrition/nutrition%20 program%20staff/whatarethediff.htm

41. Who are physical therapists (PTs)? (2010). APTA.org. Retrieved May 4, 2012 from http://www.apta.org.

42. Becker, B. (2005). *Physical Medicine and Rehabilitation: Principles and Practice,* (4th, Vol. 1. pp. 479-492). Philadelphia: Lippincott Williams and Wilkins.

43. Haglund L. (2003). Concepts in Occupational Therapy. *Occupational Therapy International*, *10*, 253-268.

44. What is a case manager? CMSA.org. Retrieved June 24, 2012, from http://www.cmsa.org.

45. Koongstvedt, P.R. (2001). "The Managed Health Care Handbook," Fourth Edition. Burlington MA: Jones & Bartlett Publishers.

46. Bluhm W.F. (2003). Group Insurance: Fourth Edition. Winstead CT. Actex Publications.

Chapter 6

1. Whelhan, F.D. (2011, January, 05). *Medicare Launches Deeply Disappointing Physician Compare Website.* Forbes.com. Retrieved April 24, 2012 *http://www.forbes.com.*
2. Stoppler, M. (2012). *How to Choose a Doctor.* Medicinenet.com. Retrieved April 2, 2012, from http://www.medicinenet.com.
3. Rabin, C. (2008, September, 29). *You Can Find Dr. Right, With Some Effort.* Nytimes.com. Retrieved April 3, 2012, from http://www.nytimes.com/2008/09/30/health/30find.html

Chapter 7

1. Hendrick, B. (2010, December, 07). *Survey Shows Americans Trust Their Doctors.* Medscape.com. Retrieved December 15, 2011 from http://www.medscape.com/viewarticle/733740.
2. Kleer E.A. Changes in surgical management resulting from case review at a breast cancer multidisciplinary tumor board. *Cancer, 107(10)",* 2346-2351.
3. Bodenheimer T. et al. (2002). Innovations in Primary Care – Patient Self-management of Chronic Disease in Primary Care. *JAMA, 288(19),* 2469-2475.

Chapter 8

1. Kohn, L. T., Corrigan, J., & Donaldson, M. S. (2000). *To err is human: Building a safer health system.* Washington, DC: National Academy Press.

2. Landrigan C.P., Parry, G.J., Bones C.B., Hackbarth A.D., Goldmann D.A., and Sharek P.J. Temporal Trends in Rates of Patient Harm Resulting from Medical Care. N Engl J Med 2010; 363:2124-2134

3. U.S. Department of Health and Human Services. Office of Inspector General. 2010. *Adverse events in hospitals: National incidence among Medicare beneficiaries.* Washington, DC: Department of Health and Human Services.

4. Jencks, S. F., Williams M. V., and Coleman E. A. (2009) Rehospitalizations among patients in the Medicare fee for-service program. *N Engl J Med,* 360(14):1418-1428.

5. Gawande, A. (2012, August 13). "Big Med." The New Yorker. Retrieved September 12, 2012 from *http://www.newyorker. com/reporting/2012/08/13/120813fa_fact_gawande*

Chapter 9

1. Tuskegee Syphilis Study Legacy Committee. (1996, May 20) "Final Report of the Tuskegee Syphilis Study Legacy Committee." Retrieved April 25, 2012 from http://www.hsl. virginia.edu/historical/medical_history/bad_blood/report. cfm.

2. Office for Human Research Protections (OHRP) (2005, June 23). "Protection of Human Subjects." *Title 45, Code of Federal Regulations, Part 46.* US Department of Health and Human Services. Retrieved December 29, 2011, from http://www. hhs.gov/ohrp/humansubjects/guidance/45cfr46.htm.

3. Understanding Clinical Trials. (2012, August). Clinicaltrials. gov. Retrieved May 4, 2013 from http://clinicaltrials.gov/ ct2/info/understand.

Chapter 10

1. Mayne L., Girod C., and Weltz S. (2012). *2012 Milliman Medical Index.* Milliman research report. Retrieved August 28, 2012 from *http://insight.milliman.com/ article.php?cntid=8078&utm_source=milliman&utm_ medium=web&utm_content=MMI-mktg&utm_ campaign=Healthcare&utm_terms=Milliman+Medical+Index.*

2. Kaiser Family Foundation. (2009). *Data Note: Americans' Satisfaction with Insurance Coverage.* Retrieved August 17, 2012 from http://www.kff.org/kaiserpolls/upload/7979.pdf.

3. Individual and Family Health Insurance FAQs. (2012). Ehealthinsurance.com. Retrieved August 19, 2012 from http://www.ehealthinsurance.com/

4. Centers for Disease Control and Prevention (2010, January 10). *Health Risk Appraisals,* CDC.gov. Retrieved July 28, 2012 from http://www.cdc.gov/nccdphp/dnpao/hwi/ programdesign/health_risk_appraisals.htm.

5. How to Home Guide; Health Costs. *(2012) How to Appeal a Health Insurance Denial.* The Wall Street Journal Online. Retrieved September 22, 2012 from **http://guides.wsj. com/health/health-costs/how-to-appeal-a-health- insurance-denial/**

6. Taking Gripes Over Insurance to the Top Brass. (2009, August 19). The Wall Street Journal. Retrieved August 12,

2012 from *http://online.wsj.com/article/SB1000142405297020 404420457435863030340569624.html*

7. How To File a Health insurance Complaint.(2010). Ebuyingguide.com. Retrieved October 1, 2012 from *http:// www.ebuyingguides.com/how/health_insurance_c.htm*

8. Flinn, R. (2012, May 21). Health Bargain Hunters Use Websites to Cut Doctor Bills. Bloomberg.com. Retrieved July 10, 2012 from http://www.bloomberg.com/news/2012-05-21/health-bargain-hunters-use-websites-to-cut-doctor-bills.html

9. Bodine, A. How to Pay Hospital Bills Without Insurance. eHow.com. Retrieved July 31, 2012 from http://www. ehow.com/how_4464666_pay-hospital-bills-insurance. html#ixzz1xAPyEcoS.

10. Paying for CAM Treatment – CAM Spending in the United States. (July 2011) NCCAM.nih.gov. Retrieved October 2, 2012 from http://nccam.nih.gov/health/financial.

Index

stress hormones, 32, 54, 64, 66, 68
stressors, 41-42, 61-62, 64
stroke, 14, 34, 40, 42, 66, 78, 80, 83, 89, 96, 111, 117-19, 156-57
support groups, 30-31, 35, 145, 168, 177
surgeons, 77, 81, 83-84
surgery, 22, 46, 74-75, 77-78, 81-83, 87, 89-91, 101, 108, 115, 128, 138, 141, 143, 155, 160, 162, 207, 213
symptom diary, 148, 150
symptoms, 20, 26-27, 30, 35, 47, 59, 96, 98-99, 104, 136, 140, 147-48, 180, 207, 257

T

tai chi, 64, 67
TCM (Traditional Chinese Medicine), 91, 99
teaching hospitals, 78, 88
television, 57
thermometer, 61
thermostat, 61
treatment plan, 32, 73, 90, 92-93, 101, 120, 133, 143, 146, 148-50, 159, 163, 167, 172
Tricare, 91
Tuskegee Syphilis Experiments, 181

U

undersleeping, 53-54
UVB (ultraviolet rays), 50-51, 250

V

vaccinations, 79, 97
vata, 102-5
vitamins, 49, 51-52, 92, 250
volunteering, 35-36, 248
vomiting, 58, 101, 113

W

water intake, 59-60
weight gain, 54
well-being, 36, 46, 72, 108-9, 144, 173-74, 178, 180
WHO (World Health Organization), 101, 249-50, 256

Y

yoga, 57, 64, 67, 105-6

ABOUT THE AUTHOR

D R. MELISSA CLARKE, a physician for over 20 years, has a passion for empowering patients with the know-how to take ownership of their healthcare. A practicing doctor, population health expert at the forefront of healthcare reform, former medical school assistant dean, and patient advocate, Dr. Clarke has a hands-on understanding of our healthcare system from all perspectives, including as a patient herself. She knows the challenges that patients face at every turn trying to get quality care, and has been able to help countless individuals overcome them. Board certified in emergency medicine, Dr. Clarke is a graduate of University of California, San Francisco School of Medicine and Harvard College. This background, coupled with a certification in acupuncture, and an extensive knowledge of alternative healthcare, makes her a supporter of integrating the best of eastern and western medicine. Dr. Clarke has been a healthcare commentator in numerous newsletters, radio and TV spots, including TV appearances on the Roland Martin Show. With a growing social media reach, she provides valuable health news and commentary designed to empower us all to take care of our most valuable resource - our health. Follow her Facebook page Dr Melissa Clarke, and on Twitter @DrMelissaClarke.

For information about this book and speaking engagements, contact her at info@drmelissaclarke.com.